Praise for *I Chose Love*

(continued from back cover)

"*I Chose Love* is a book about real willpower when all odds are against you. When all others say 'No you can't' or 'There is nothing we can do,' you keep going until you find an answer. It is truly a book about beating the odds and facing fears that you never knew you had with fearlessness and raw determination."

—Jamie M. Lee, DNM, IMD

"After the devastating diagnosis of an inoperable brain tumor, Sandi steadily found her way into forming a trusting friendship with her own body. With her life at stake, she had the courage to see her life and relationships with clarity and to set boundaries. She knew she had to be on her own side, and she let that be her guide in dealing with a frustrating patronizing medical system and dysfunctional personal relationships. Each chapter concludes with nuggets of advice and encouragement. Sandi's life now reflects her hard-won wisdom."

—Lynn Fraser, Founder, Stillpoint Method of Healing Trauma

"Sandi Gold proudly recounts a life story that is not only inspirational, but motivates the reader to journey through life in a similar, upbeat way. Which is, facing each danger, challenge and blind corner with a higher state-of-consciousness, that's truly transformative. Her ability from page 1 to engender empathy and point the reader to the notion that 'love is the answer' is transcendent in its delivery. In short, this book is a *sine qua non* for any household, and is *so*, so good at suggesting what the human heart too often lacks: real hope, and the way to find it. Read this 'victorious living' account, and you'll wonder why you didn't see these tailor-made solutions before."

—Greg W. Kay, U.S. Diplomatic Corps, Retired. Future author of
A Christian, a Gay Guy and a Diplomat Walk into a Bar...

I Chose Love

I Chose Love

How to Thrive After a Life-Threatening Illness
Using Love to Guide You

By Sandi Gold

For my mother, Margaret

Table of Contents

Acknowledgments

I could not have possibly had the success in healing if it had not been for my mother who is responsible for my never-say-die spirit, something that we both share. The threat of losing a child is one of the worst things any parent can experience. My mother fought with all the strength she had—sometimes alongside me and sometimes against, after her fears hijacked and overwhelmed her. I will always deeply love and appreciate her in a way that only a daughter can love her mother. I also want to acknowledge my brother and sister for being who they are, because if it weren't for them, I wouldn't be the person I am today.

I certainly never would have had been able to complete this book if I had not had the all the help I had from so many people, but especially from Susan Adams, Karen Rand Anderson, LeNae Atkinson, Joe Azar, Rosemarie Balcom, Rose Bednar, Oshea Bills, Lynn Brallier, Theresa Broach, Diane Brown, Van Brown, Victoria Burdick, Stacy Collette, Geoff Constantine, Lois Constantine, Ruth Crocker, Donna Darmody, Marilyn Dayton, Julianne Eanniello, Linda Evans, David Farland, Susan Fox, Lynn Fraser, Hollie Galloway, Barbara Ganim, BJ Gaynor, Greg Gersch, Ann Grimes, Alexis Heitman, Laura Hopkins, Priscilla Humphrey, Kathy Izbicki, Cathy Johansen, Palin John, David Johnson, Greg Kay, Bruce Kerzner, Scott Kiloby, Paul Kuhn, Jamie Lee, Lori Leyden, Sarah Lucas, Angela MacLeod, Marlisa McLaughlin, Hillary Oat, Dan O'Connor, Deirdre O'Connor, Bill McNichols, Gail Hooker Mills, Patrick Newton, Todd and Elaine Patterson, Jane Percy, Breck Perkins, Kathryn Haddock Petaja, Alicia Piccolo, Victoria Pitt, Connie Plessman, Lillian Poston, Janice Prentice, Michael Rauh, Gainor Roberts, Kimmie Ross, Kelly Russell-Presley, Sharon Miller Schaffer, Polly Seip, Divya Sharma, Bernie Siegel, Ginger Smyle, Stephen Trelli, Rhonda Tyler, Juuso Voltti, Beth Walker, Sherry Walker, Robin & Jon Western, Caitlin Wheeler, Karin Forde Whittemore, Carol Zeilman, and everyone else that I regretfully forgot.

Foreword by Fr. William Hart McNichols

Keep a good heart. That's the most important thing in life.
It's not how much money you make or what you can acquire.
The art of it is to keep a good heart.
—Joni Mitchell

Sandi and I met in a drawing class at Boston University in September of 1971. I was a young Catholic seminarian studying for the priesthood, taking philosophy courses at Boston College. At that time, they were lacking in any visual arts program, so I took art classes three times a week at BU.

I had only recently moved to Boston and really knew no one. Being rather shy and introverted I was hoping to slip in and out of class unnoticed. But Sandi joyfully ran over to my art bench, while I was working, and said to the whole class "Oh look what he's drawing!" And everyone did. I turned as white as the drawing paper, and then, quickly bright red because that astute "intervention" ended my anonymity ... and that's how we became friends.

Sandi intuitively sensed my painful state of loneliness, and I think quite unconsciously wanted to bring me into human communion. That's just one little vignette about how perceptive Sandi was and is; how deeply loving and concerned for others.

Let me start right off with an understatement: this is a really good book. In fact, it's a great book. And though I've been friends with Sandi for over 50 years, and was aware of some of what she was going through, this book came as a surprise to me and even as a shock because Sandi is not one to complain. Much of what she's written she shared with no one.

We often hear about Joseph Campbell's theory of the hero's journey. Well, with this incredible autobiographical tale, Sandi takes us on a real heroine's journey. Her own story is of a nearly miraculous healing, dramatic escapes from uncaring or oblivious caregivers, and wonderful "messenger-angel-like" men and women who came just in time to offer emotional and practical help.

You'll also find in reading this book that Sandi is one of the best teachers you'll ever meet. She gives you a host of serious medical, very wise emotional, and sometimes hilarious information, in a natural and easy way to ponder and comprehend. And her constantly uplifting humor is one of her most attractive, useful, and compassionate gifts.

She is also a great artist, in the fullest sense of that word, her whole life is an art, not only as a survivor but as someone who in the midst of some terribly harrowing circumstances, still manages to bring us her considerable artistic gifts.

Because she is also beautiful on the outside too—I used to nudge her as the young men all over the BU campus would turn their heads in wonder—and yet she never really even noticed. She brings her gifts with that same lovely elegance. She brings that "mythic elixir"—as Joseph Campbell describes as that hard won, yet very simple, healing experience for others who too may be feeling alone and separated from the rest of the world. She's been on a journey that few have been on and has come back to share her hard-earned gift of healing to anyone who will receive it.

What a privilege it is for me to introduce to you my dear friend Sandi. I know full well she'll most naturally change your life too.

Fr. William Hart McNichols
Albuquerque, New Mexico
Internationally known iconographer and co-author with Christopher Pramuk of the forthcoming book from Orbis Press, *All My Eyes See: The Artistic Vocation of Fr. William Hart McNichols*

Foreword with Dr. Bernie Siegel

I am convinced that unconditional love is the most powerful
known stimulant of the immune system. The truth is: love heals.
—Dr. Bernie Siegel, *Love, Medicine and Miracles*

"You are a survivor and thriver," Bernie Siegel wrote in an email to me. I leaped from my chair and cheered! Bernie's book *Love, Medicine and Miracles* was published in 1986, just months before I was told I had six months to a year to live. He reinforced my belief in the healing power of love at the absolutely perfect time. And I don't think this was a coincidence. Often I would "arm" myself by carrying his book to doctor's appointments (though it wasn't until about ten years later that any doctor ever asked about it.)

I met Bernie (as he prefers to be called) in 1994 after articles written about me appeared in *The New York Times, People Magazine, The Boston Globe*, and in numerous other papers across the country. I was interviewed by Susan Stamberg on NPR. And ABC's news show *20/20* filmed me after I painted and erased a 63' mural to depict the importance of appreciating our lives while we are still alive. As my way of thanking Bernie for the contribution he made to my life and for the person he is, I used the attention I was receiving to highlight him.

In his email he asked that I share this with you: "Remember most of all, if you recover when it was unexpected by your doctor, you did not have a spontaneous remission. You had a self-induced healing due to the transformation, like a caterpillar breaking out of his cocoon and becoming a butterfly."

He also sent me the following examples on the power of love to heal.

- A study of Harvard undergraduates revealed that those who felt unloved by their parents were 98% more likely to have a serious illness by the time they reached middle age, versus 24% of those who believed that their parents loved them.

- A woman named Evy was diagnosed with an advanced form of A.L.S. and told she had about six months to live. Because she had polio as a child, she also had withered limbs. She went home and sat naked in her wheelchair in front of her mirror. She made a list of all the ways she hated her body and her life—and she allowed herself to feel all this pain. Every day she forgave those she needed to forgive. At the end of each 20-minute session, she wrote at least one positive thing about herself. This list of her good qualities gradually grew until she only felt love and compassion for herself. She saw herself as the loving woman she was created to be. Eventually she not only walked again, but Evy became the first person to completely recover from A.L.S.

- Disappointed that he missed the funeral of a patient who had gone to Colorado to die in the mountains, Bernie called to ask the family why they hadn't notified him of the funeral. But his patient answered the phone and told Bernie, "It was so beautiful I forgot to die."

- A lawyer whose parents wanted him to be a lawyer and not a violinist, closed his law office when he developed cancer. He got a job playing his violin in an orchestra, and he didn't die as expected.

Bernie also wanted me to share with you, "Those who have pets have a lower death rate and women's death rate is lower than men. It is about relationships. And not about doing something."

Bernie wrote that I could use what he wrote as I so desire and to integrate it into what I write and to use both our names.

So delightfully I am signing this with love from both of us.

Bernie Siegel and Sandi Gold

Introduction

After I received a call from my neurologist telling me I had an inoperable, fast growing, life-threatening brain tumor, I was sent to the hospital. Here I was greeted by uncomfortable smiles as each technician efficiently performed her job. Test after test was conducted as my fears and tension grew. During my overnight stay not even a social worker was assigned to discuss the elephant in the room.

After I was discharged, I saw four more neurologists to get their opinions. Each told me the same thing—I had six months to a year to live. I saw these doctors in December 1986 through January 1987 and yet I am still very much alive.

The responsibility of finding a way to keep myself alive fell upon my shoulders. I decided that every one of these neurologists was thinking too myopically. I refused to be restricted by what they believed. Instead, I chose to use the strongest form of energy that's ever existed to save my life. I chose love.

There's a reason we are born with a desire to be loved and a need to share our love with others. When newborn babies struggling to live are held, their survival rates increase dramatically. Haven't we all felt this loving, supportive, and healing energy that is transferred when someone is attentive to our needs? As adults, most of us become energized when we fall in love. We know what it feels like as two uplifting vibrational energies align, intensify, and enhance each other. We all know—whether we are on the giving or receiving end—that love affects us and all our lives.

So why is using love to heal our bodies such a foreign concept to our medical system? Why, when I was in the hospital, did not one person ask how I was coping after I was told I was dying just hours before?

Because of this bizarre and troublesome experience, I wanted nothing more to do with the sterile, detached, and cold way I was treated. Nor did

1

I appreciate how discourteous my neurologist was to me just days later because he falsely believed I wasn't telling him all my symptoms.

This is why, just weeks after my diagnosis, I decided that however much time I had left to live, I would use love to guide me through the arduous months or years ahead.

In my highly sensitive state, I began to notice that whenever I encountered a problem or conflict, my body contracted in fear. I could feel my tightened muscles restrict love's energy from freely flowing. Because I could feel this weaken my body, it felt like a threat to my life. Over time, whenever I felt fear, I taught myself to form the habit of focusing on the love in my heart.

Teaching myself to live with an open heart had unexpected benefits: not only did this allow me to feel more love and strengthen me, but I also became a more patient, forgiving, compassionate, and loving person. As I learned to trust more, my body relaxed. This allowed me to think more clearly and see that I had options.

Our body is our most loyal, loving, and supportive friend. It never stops trying to communicate and help us. It's amazing how magnificent our bodies have been designed, and how wise and knowledgeable they truly are. And they never lie to us. They always tell the truth.

I taught myself to become somatically oriented and learn the language my body speaks. I fine-tuned my ability to understand it by carefully listening and respecting everything my body said.

Have you noticed the effect your thoughts have on your body? When you see a policeman in your car's rear-view mirror, you can often feel your heart beating faster, which proves our bodies are not just physical. Yet while I was in the hospital, my doctors only focused on my physical body. Thankfully, I knew that this wasn't enough; that this was too restrictive and wasn't going to save my life.

I learned, like every other child is taught in school, that Einstein discovered how all matter in the universe is energy vibrating at various frequencies. I knew my body was energy too, and the highest form of energy is love, and that this was what was missing from my medical care.

In this book I clearly show what I did—step by step—after I was told my life would soon end. I explain how I aligned myself with love to strengthen myself and how I used my love and the love and care that people generously gave me to better attune myself to my body's wisdom. And I also share how I learned to cope with negative, draining, and unsupportive energy that I encountered that felt life threatening at the time to me.

I also reveal some of my embarrassing behavior to help you understand that perfection is not required. If I can help you avoid some of the painful pitfalls that I experienced, I am more than willing to show how silly and even ridiculous I acted at times.

Because we are all individuals, my goal is not to convince you to do what I did. Rather, I have shared as accurately as I can both what I did and why I did it to help you follow and understand my process. I hope this book will inspire you to expand your thinking and help you decide what is most appropriate for you and give you a healthier and happier life.

I am not claiming to know the only way a person can heal themselves. I am simply sharing what worked for me after I had to find a way to stay alive. I am encouraging you to find your own way because this will be the best and most effective way for you.

In this book, I share not only what I learned about love's healing capabilities, but how using love as my guide not only improved my health when I was struggling, but improved me as a person and my entire life.

1

Even Cockroaches Can be Beneficial

If anyone were to tell me that hundreds of cockroaches scurrying up their kitchen wall helped to save their life, I wouldn't have believed them. But a fast-growing, inoperable, life-threatening brain tumor was discovered before it had a chance to kill me thanks to these apocalypse-surviving intruders.

I was doing all the cleaning, grocery shopping, laundry, cooking, and washing the dishes for a month after I moved in with my boyfriend Gary. And, just like him, I had a full-time job. I was miserable, exhausted, and feeling disillusioned because he wouldn't help with any of the housework. I told him I was moving out unless we went to counseling. To my surprise, Pamela, our new "marriage" therapist, said that *my* behavior wasn't healthy. If I wanted Gary to do the dishes, I had to stop washing them.

"And he purposely kept me from knowing he smoked dope every day the whole time we dated. I grew up around people with addictions, so I've never wanted anything to do with them. How can I trust him now?" I asked.

Pamela said, "For me to agree to counsel you, you must agree to never discuss Gary's drug use again. Not with him. Not with me. Never. His smoking is his decision and if you don't like it, you can move out. The only way you'll know you can trust him to do the dishes is to give him a chance. Stop washing them."

Dirty dishes piled up in our kitchen. I was appalled that anyone would expect me to live like this and that Gary would allow himself to live in such filth. He'd been using dope as an avoidance tactic for over half his life. He didn't seem to care how the dishes affected me.

Because relationships are mirrors that reveal and expose us, after I moved in with him, Gary found it impossible to accept what our relationship disclosed about him. He had never lived with a woman before, and I believe this intimacy (meaning into-me-see) was just too foreign and frightening for him. It made him feel too vulnerable. Because he had smoked dope since he was young, it interfered with his ability to learn how to cope effectively with his emotions. He then resented me for the discomfort he felt and decided I had to be controlled.

Pamela had instructed me to say nothing about the dishes, but respect whatever choice Gary made: "He's a grown man and he has a right to make decisions for himself."

My energy had been rapidly declining ever since I had moved in with Gary. I was scared and desperate to feel like myself again, so I followed Pamela's instructions and said nothing about my home looking like a place the health department would condemn. After six days, I was carrying our dirty dinner plates to the kitchen. I flicked on the overhead lights using my right shoulder and froze as a dark pulsating mass containing hundreds of cockroaches scurried to escape the bright light.

In an out-of-control frenzy and with all my strength, I smashed every dirty dish I saw, releasing months of pent-up frustration as I was forced to accept that I had been snookered: Gary wasn't the man he pretended to be the entire year we dated.

"Why are you torturing me? What did I ever do but love you in every possible way I knew?" I yelled between sobs.

I only stopped crying when the phone rang, and Gary didn't answer it. Where was he? Hiding like a frightened child?

"Hello, Sandi. It's your mutha," my mother playfully said. "I'm calling because—" I wailed into the phone before she could finish. I explained how horrible Gary had been acting and how unhappy I was. It was rare for me to complain to my mother about anything. I loved her dearly, but she had a tendency to get too involved. Respecting others' boundaries was not something she did.

"Hormonal problems run in our family. Your sister is having problems, too. Call a gynecologist in the morning," was her motherly advice.

Believing I had severe PMS (premenstrual syndrome) that was giving me a temper, I made an appointment the next day. After a short examination, the gynecologist sent me to a neurologist who sent me to a clinic to be tested right away.

The Importance of Speaking Up for Yourself

As the dishes piled up, I was forced to see the reality of my relation-ship. Refusing to tolerate Gary's behavior any longer was an act of self-love. Because I spoke up for myself, I didn't die, and the brain tumor was discovered before it could end my life.

Notice how often your body talks to you—telling you when you need rest, that you're hungry, that you are too cold or hot. Notice how it's always to your advantage to listen. Notice how your body is a loyal, supportive, and loving friend. It never lies and you can always trust it.

At the end of every chapter, there is a place for you to journal, as you can see in the space below. Start here by keeping a list of the helpful ways your body assists you, and the times you did and didn't listen. List the advantages you gained when you listened, and what it cost you when you didn't.

_____

_____

_____

_____

_____

_____

_____

_____

_____

_____

_____

_____

_____

_____

_____

_____

_____

2

When You Feel You're Losing Control

"Do I eat fish?" I asked, thinking perhaps I had heard the question wrong because people at the clinic were talking and Christmas carols were playing overhead.

"If you eat fish, you most likely won't get nauseous from the iodine in the drip I'm about to put in your arm," a young technician explained, while rolling up my shirt sleeve.

"Oh. Yes, I love fish."

Being in the heart of Washington D.C., space must have been limited because the CT scan machine I had been instructed to lie beside was situated in a corner of this clinic's waiting room.

I thought the stress of moving in with Gary had exacerbated my PMS, but the gynecologist I had just seen this morning questioned this and sent me to see a neurologist right away. When he asked me to walk from heel to toe, I lost my balance. The doctor thought I might have had a stroke and said I needed to be tested immediately, which was why I was there.

While I was lying on my back beside the CT scan machine, I studied the mustard-colored water stains on the ceiling to help soothe my nerves. I also eavesdropped on the conversation of the people seated closest to me. A mother was attempting to calm her son. He responded in that annoying teenage tone, saying he wanted to go home and "forget about seeing this stupid doctor." Farther from me, a young couple debated where they would have dinner later that night. He wanted Mexican food. She wanted Chinese. Mexican sounded good to me, and I hoped Gary would be amenable.

After the test was completed, I was just starting to relax when the entire room went silent, as if a light switch had been flipped. I was scared and perplexed until, leaning over from behind my head, the technician whispered that my neurologist was on the phone and pointed to the receptionist's office.

Unconcealed fear was what I saw in the crowd of staring faces as I walked across the room. The receptionist's office was empty, void of all life. Standing behind the sliding glass window that anyone could open at any time to announce their arrival, I felt exposed and vulnerable before I even picked up the phone.

"Hello," I said. "This is Sandi."

"I'm sorry to have to tell you this, Ms. Gold, but you have a hemangioblastoma in the pons section of your brain."

Glancing up to distract myself, I was startled to see Gary step from the elevator and walk towards me. When I'd called to update him in between appointments, he hadn't asked if I wanted him here. He just assumed I did, though it was sweet he wanted to come and support me.

Gary looked surprised to see me standing where the receptionist sits. Keeping my eyes glued on his, I used a stern, unwelcoming expression to signal that things were not good. He responded by grinning back, twisting his mouth, making goofy faces, and crossing his eyes like small children do, while I struggled to hear my doctor.

"A hemangioblastoma is a fast-growing tumor, but because of its location, there's no way we can operate. It's life-threatening, but there's nothing we can do for you."

Gary still grinned playfully, lost in his own little world. *Dear Lord. He's got to be stoned.*

As the distance between us diminished, I felt pressure building. To put an end to his obliviousness, I extended my right hand in front of me and gave him the universal thumbs-down gesture, and watched as his expression turned to terror. *Stop feeling, Sandi. You've got to stay strong.*

"Hello? Ms. Gold? Are you still there?"

"I'm here. So, we'll talk later," I shot back and hung up the phone.

Lowering my head and using my long blonde hair to shield my face, I ran to catch the elevator, stopping only briefly to grab my winter coat and small black purse. From somewhere behind me, Gary shouted, insisting that I wait for him. Never had I turned my back and run from him before, so why didn't he understand why I was running away now?

"Tell me what the doctor said," Gary demanded after he caught up to me by the elevator.

Whenever Gary got aggressive, I took a deep breath, just like I had trained myself to do to keep from losing my temper, before I whispered, "I have a brain tumor."

Leaning my face close to his, I looked at him with that wide-eyed stare that most people know means, "I really can't talk now, so don't you dare push me."

"What? You've got to tell me everything the doctor said. Come on, Sandi."

Dear God. Please get him to back off.

"Stop playing games!" Gary shouted.

I can't even have my own reaction after being told I'm going to die without him making this about him too?

"The doctor wants me to go to the hospital tomorrow, but I really can't say anything else. Just wait until we get outside. Please."

"Tell me what the doctor said now!"

By the grace of God, the elevator came. Carefully, we wedged our way in and turned our backs on the strangers packed inside this small container. Despite the warm air smelling of sweat, I tried to calm myself by taking long, slow, deep breaths until Gary grabbed me by my upper arm.

"Tell me what the doctor said."

Like air escaping from a punctured balloon, my anger claimed its freedom and liberated itself.

"I have a f@#king brain tumor!"

Gary froze, along with everyone else surrounding me.

"It's in the pons section of my brain, wherever the hell that is. They can't operate because it's too risky. It's fast-growing and I'm to check into the hospital tomorrow, but I don't know why. If they can't do anything, why can't they leave me alone? Why can't you?"

Silence. Everyone avoided looking at me. As we slowly descended, I listened to a faint electrical humming sound coming from somewhere inside the elevator shaft. I zeroed in on a single soft click that indicated every floor we passed. Finally, we reached the ground level, and the doors slid open. I entered a different world where my life would forever be transformed.

Over the previous ten years, about a half dozen doctors had misdiagnosed me as having PMS. I was told again and again that I could control it using various suggested remedies, but I couldn't. I felt like a failure. I lost respect for myself as my patience wore thin. Just months earlier, I'd developed a temper and become someone I didn't like. Using the same strategy I used as a child to feel safe at home, I was extra kind and loving to Gary, but he was extremely controlling, and insisted that I think and act like him.

I moved to Washington, D.C. when I was 28. Five years later, I moved in with Gary, believing we would marry and start a family. But we fought on our very first evening living together after I discovered he hadn't been honest with me. Though I tried in every way I knew, this argument never got resolved.

"I've smoked every day since I was 13, and I'm not stopping just because you've got a problem. I even passed the law boards while stoned, so stop acting so ridiculous," he said that night.

I had spoken up for myself and expressed my perspective. I told him that his constant smoking made me very nervous. Gary got so furious, he frightened me. I ran and locked myself in the bathroom. Because I wouldn't unlock the door as he demanded, he removed the doorknob, swung the door open, and leaned against the doorframe and grinned as he watched me cry.

When someone starts using drugs as a teenager to avoid the pain from their childhood, their brains develop differently. Their emotional skills are underdeveloped. Though he was an outstanding lawyer who skillfully resolved intricate legal problems, whenever he felt threatened by me, the only thing he knew was to intimidate. When he came to the clinic to support me, my diagnosis had threatened the poor man, so he couldn't be supportive even if he wanted. The real problem was, because he lacked self-awareness and he never tried to see things from my perspective, he never saw the harm that he was doing.

Be True to Yourself and Treat Yourself Lovingly

Rather than putting additional stress on myself by worrying about the test results, as an act of self-love, I entertained myself by looking at water stains on the ceiling and eavesdropping on people's conversations. When I wasn't ready to talk about my prognosis, I defended and protected myself. Be true to yourself and treat yourself with love and respect.

Write down the ways that you are true to yourself and treat yourself lovingly.

_____

_____

_____

_____

_____

_____

_____

_____

_____

Write down the times you did not. In what ways might you treat yourself better? And in what ways has not being true or good to yourself cost you?

_____

_____

_____

_____

_____

_____

_____

3

Trust How You Respond

Neither Gary nor I said a word after we exited the elevator and walked out of the building. In the middle of the unpaved parking lot, Gary suddenly stopped short, and I crashed into the back of him. My head must have been lowered because I can still picture what the ground looked like. It had hard-packed, sand-colored soil with patches of small stones scattered about.

"I have a meeting I'm supposed to be at. You drove yourself here, so we have two cars. You can drive yourself home, can't you?" Gary said.

My drive home began alright because I only had to follow the two red taillights on Gary's brown Honda, but when his car turned away from the direction of our home, I panicked. I assumed the plan was *after* he saw me safely home, he would go to his meeting.

All I have to do is drive. Just drive, Sandi.

I was completely on my own now, in the dark, in rush hour traffic in downtown Washington, D.C. It started to rain and the reflections on the wet pavement from the oncoming headlights strained my eyes.

As if I was floating, it felt like my little red Sentra alternated from having three to four tires on the road. I didn't associate this with just being told I had a life-threatening brain tumor or with Gary's unexpected disappearing act. I was probably too scared to think about this.

Gary had to go to his meeting. It's important that he be there. All I need to do is drive. Just drive, Sandi.

At the clinic, I had responded from the reptilian part of my brain, which controls self-preservation to ensure our survival. My body released additional adrenaline to protect me after Gary kept trying to stop me, which made thinking and driving more difficult. By grabbing my arm in the elevator and demanding I do as he said, because this felt threatening, I had instinctively entered into the fight phase.

The slow-motion floating sensation I felt while I was driving was me dropping into the freeze phase as my body went into shock. Using mind-over-matter, something I had done since childhood, I was able to slow this down.

I was about eight years old, sitting in the bleachers with my mother, watching my brother's Little League game, when a hard-hit line drive hit my right upper thigh.

"Sandi! Sandi! Sandi!" my mother shouted as she leaped to her feet.

No siree, I wasn't about to break our family rule—don't ever upset Mom. I stood and widely grinned.

Spectators from both teams applauded as I blushed. Over the speaker, a male voice announced that a free hot dog was waiting at the concession stand for me because I demonstrated "such impressive bravery for a little girl." Bravery? Doesn't everyone strive to protect their mother from going off her rocker? If our mother's melodrama disrupted my siblings in any way, they would have made life impossible for me.

Responding as I did when the baseball hit my thigh was like me refusing to go into shock while I drove myself home. Just as I had protected my mother, I never told Gary how difficult driving was. I told him some things about the drive while laughing to keep things light because I didn't know how much more stress he could handle and when he would reach his limit.

Almost a decade passed before I realized how inappropriate it had been for Gary to leave me at the clinic. If I couldn't see that I deserved to be seen safely home after I was diagnosed with a life-threatening brain tumor, I wondered how many other countless ways had I compromised myself? And how many people had taken advantage of me?

The next day, I reluctantly checked into the hospital thinking, *if they can't do anything for me, what's the point?*

I hated having the angiogram test because a catheter was pushed into a blood vessel on the right side of my groin to allow my doctors to look at my brain. Because this wound could easily get infected, the right half of my pubic area had to be shaved. I had a brain tumor, so my pubic hair was shaved? I wasn't in the least bit amused.

To avoid infection, once this test was completed, I had to keep my right leg straight and rest in bed for eight hours. Every hour some stranger entered my room, lifted a white washcloth covering my privates (which no longer were), and studied my new tiny pink wound. Trying to sleep with my leg straight and having my privates continually examined put me in a foul mood. Just as I succeeded in falling asleep, like a mother duck with her baby chicks in tow, a doctor led a group of young, eager interns into my room. And they awakened me, so I didn't smile to welcome them.

The doctor looked like he could have been Woody Allen's attractive younger brother. He was dark-haired, small-boned, and in his mid to late fifties. He smiled as he walked past my bed and politely introduced himself and his restless students. By the way he nonchalantly grabbed a brown wooden clipboard from my bedpost to read about my case, I could tell he had been teaching for many years.

As he stretched his arm and turned his body, I read his name tag: Dr. Horowitz, Neurosurgeon. Reading this excited me. I had a neurosurgeon just appear in my room! Smiling graciously, I now scanned the room to welcome all my visitors.

My state of health is about to be discussed among this doctor's entourage. Something might be said that could save my life, I thought until I saw the blood drain from the doctor's face as he pushed his shoulders back and stood more erect in an attempt to look calm and cool.

"Go on ahead to the next room," he told his students, waving his right hand in the air in a butterfly-like fashion to encourage their rapid exit.

Stunned and disappointed, I watched as the students left with the doctor following closely behind. Unwilling to miss this serendipitous opportunity, I yelled, "Talk to me! Please."

With his hand still grasping the doorknob, the doctor froze.

Had I offended him? But I was just told I would die.

In the upper left-hand corner of the room, on the opposite side of my bed from where the doctor was playing statue, I heard a noise. I turned to see what it was. As my eyes crossed the room, I saw four sharply defined rays of light shining through four large windows. Seeing this ethereal beauty took my breath away.

Inside each ray, thousands of tiny floating particles danced about in slow-motion. This spellbinding moment hypnotized me until I remembered where I was. I continued to look to my left and discovered the noise I had heard was Gary shuffling his feet as he awakened from a nap. I turned my head back to the right and saw that the doctor had not moved.

Realizing he must be waiting for me to speak, I said, "My neurologist thinks my tumor is inoperable and quickly growing. He's pretty much told me I'm going to die. What do you think?"

He turned, looked me in the eyes and gently smiled before he said, "Your timing is good because of the recent invention of the MRI. In another year or so, we may have something that could help you."

"Really? A year from now? Do you really think I'll be alive a year from now?"

An awkward pause followed. "No," he said. "But I can tell you there's a doctor doing something at Massachusetts General Hospital in Boston that might be able to help you." He didn't know this doctor's name, but he knew a doctor who worked in the same hospital who would know. His name was Dr. Ojemann.

Dr. Horowitz was the first person who reacted to my diagnosis in a caring, earnest manner. He hadn't been afraid to show his emotions, which revealed what a remarkable man he was and that he could be trusted.

I felt bad for causing him discomfort, but my goal was to live. And I had to do whatever I could to accomplish this. Because I spoke up for myself, this was the first time I heard of something that might save my life. A nurse came into my room and the doctor silently slipped away to join his waiting students.

The next morning, being discharged from the hospital felt wrong and disjointed. Except for Dr. Horowitz, who just happened to walk in my room, no one offered me any help or encouragement. No one was made available to talk with me. It felt like my health problem was too dangerous for even the staff to discuss. And this only made it even more frightening for me.

It didn't feel safe to go home. The day before I hadn't wanted to come to the hospital, but now I could feel my resistance to leaving. Even before my diagnosis, I hadn't felt safe living with Gary, especially since Pamela, our counselor, had just told me he couldn't be trusted.

While waiting for him to pick me up, I heard what sounded like a series of switches systematically turning off inside my head. An invisible veil fell over me, separating me from the rest of the world or perhaps protecting me from Gary, who had just arrived to drive me home.

Ever since our first argument, if I ever caused him any discomfort, if I simply expressed a perspective that differed from his, he got angry and yelled. The more I tried to explain myself, the angrier he got. He had even become upset a few weeks before because I hadn't liked a movie we saw together.

"When I take you to a movie, I want you to enjoy it," he said, not caring how macho he was acting.

I was treated as being wrong for just being me, so I couldn't tell him how scared I was or that I felt weak and light-headed. This would make Gary uncomfortable, and things would only get worse for me.

He was silent on the way home. Was he sighing heavily because he wanted me to see how stressed he was and that he wasn't going to stick around much longer? Or was he just being his manipulative self, trying to get me to feel sorry for him? To help reinforce him, to give him strength, I would have to praise him, express my gratitude often, and tell him that he was my hero.

"Thank you for picking me up, Gary. I don't know what I would do without you. "He dropped me off on the sidewalk in front of our home and quickly returned to work. I spent the afternoon alone, lost in thought. I had given away the last 24 hours of my life doing everything I was told, but what had I gotten in return? Having the results from these tests was important, but not as important as me keeping strong.

Allowing patients to leave the hospital feeling as invisible and insignificant as I felt wasn't healthy or right. Maybe the social worker had somehow forgotten to come see me? Someone had clearly dropped the ball. Thank God for Dr. Horowitz. If I had fallen asleep and hadn't shouted out to him, I would have felt even worse than I did.

"We fall ill, and our illness falls under the hard hand of science," Anne Boyer wrote in her book, *Undying*, published 31 years after my hospital stay, after I had the mind-blowing discovery that the hospital's most vulnerable patients' needs were inhumanly overlooked.

I told myself that just because others may fail us, whether we're sick or not, I must remember my true value and treat myself well. By honoring ourselves and the individuals we are, and not apologizing for having needs, we strengthen ourselves and our ability to live—literally.

I used to refuse help even when I needed it because I didn't want to inconvenience anyone. And I feared showing my vulnerable side. Over time, I learned it was important to admit when I needed help. I would never have lived otherwise. I had no idea what other people did after they were told they were going to die. I only know how I reacted and how I spent my first day home.

Most people think being told I had a life-threatening brain tumor would have been my biggest concern, but it wasn't. What disturbed me most was the heartless policy of the hospital—a place I associated with helping people. I had been discharged and left to fend for myself. How could anyone treat me like this? I needed help more than I ever did and this was all that I was given?

What no doubt contributed to my fears and disgust was that Pamela had recently told me that Gary had been strategically using me to his own advantage ever since I'd moved in with him.

"All his life Gary has had little control, so he's now thoroughly enjoying taking yours from you. You've been paying for his problems from his past with your blood, sweat, and tears, and anything else he can take from you."

My relationship was even worse than I thought.

"Gary doesn't care about how much pain you've been in," Pamela continued. "He got you to move in and pay half his rent when his best friend wanted your apartment. And you're cooking, cleaning, and doing his laundry. He knows he can't control his parents, so he's controlling you to make himself feel powerful."

I had a life-threatening brain tumor, and in addition to staying alive, I had to figure out a way to feel safe while living with someone I couldn't trust?

How did the hospital know I wasn't going to slash my wrists or jump in front of the Metro? They just assumed that everyone took being told they were dying in stride and didn't need help, other than being tested? They couldn't know how every patient would react. Did they really just not care?

Why wasn't there a protocol in place to assist someone in my position? Wasn't it common knowledge that being told we were going to die was difficult to hear? So why would a hospital do nothing but test me?

How had I got myself in this position? How many patients, in response to the hospital's thoughtlessness, had committed suicide? Stop! I had to figure out a way to make my illness as easy as possible for Gary.

Being sick could actually make our relationship stronger. Since we had to work as a team, this could bring us closer together. I just had to figure out how to stop Gary from wanting to take advantage of me and draining me of energy or I wasn't going to have the strength to overcome the brain tumor.

Give Yourself the Support You Need

By reassuring myself while driving, I successfully stopped myself from going into shock. And I took advantage of a neurologist entering my hospital room by asking him what ideas he had. I knew I deserved better and needed more than the hospital offered. I trusted myself and decided that especially when others fail me, I must remember my true value and treat myself with love and respect.

Write down the ways you speak up and lovingly support yourself.

_____

_____

_____

_____

_____

_____

_____

_____

Write down times when you didn't support yourself that you now regret. What did this cost you? What could you have done differently to be more supportive of yourself?

_____

_____

_____

_____

_____

_____

_____

4

We Each Have to Find Our Own Way

I called as soon as Dr. Ojemann's office opened on Monday morning. His receptionist said he wasn't available.

"I'm going to have to keep calling and make a real pest of myself until I speak to him because I was just told I could die in six months," I replied.

"I understand, but don't call back tomorrow. He's flying to D.C."

"D.C.?! Great! That's where I live. I'll pick him up at the airport and take him wherever he wants to go. Just tell me what flight he'll be on."

Laughing at my tenacity, the receptionist put me on hold. When she returned, she said the doctor would be happy to look at my pictures. I cheered and thanked her profusely.

By taking control and achieving success my first time at bat, I got my control back for the first time since I was diagnosed. Savoring this glorious moment, I basked in my victory and allowed my confidence to skyrocket. No one could stop me now and no one had better try because feeling like I did at this very moment was the fuel I needed to stay alive.

I leaped up onto my living room couch and jumped up and down like a little kid. "And I'm going to keep calling back again and again until I speak to the doctor. Because this is my life, babe, and I'm not giving up!" I shouted at the top of my lungs. Buster and Charlie, our two cats, had been sunning themselves by our large picture window. When they heard me shout, they jumped in the air simultaneously before scurrying from the room.

Later that week, after seeing my neurologist, I couldn't stop thinking about the way he had spoken to me. He had accused me of not telling him all my symptoms. He even asked Gary what I was withholding while

I was sitting there. He was treating me like a naughty little girl who was lying to him.

This doctor had never seen anyone's body react to having a brain tumor in the pons the way my body was, so he falsely concluded that I was holding back information from him. His narrow way of thinking triggered me, no doubt reminding me of Gary.

Despite playing a major role in both of these relationships, these two men acted as if what they believed was all that mattered. If my doctor had accepted that what I said was true, he wouldn't have become so exasperated and been so rude and dismissive.

"If my body is reacting the way it is, then this is how my body reacts," I tried to explain, but he kept insisting that I fit into some kind of template that he devised. Because my body didn't, he made agitated faces throughout my appointment, twisting his lips from side to side, and rolling his eyes in disgust. I tried to help him expand his myopic thinking, but I might as well have been talking to an artichoke.

After we left his office, I told Gary how frustrated I felt being treated like this, especially as a woman.

"I liked him," was all he said, as if how I felt wasn't worth discussing.

I now knew that my body was handling the tumor well, even if my doctor didn't believe this. I decided that he didn't have the necessary tools to understand my needs, but that another doctor would. Once I was able, I only used this doctor to schedule tests I needed.

No matter how great a doctor is, we live in our bodies 24 hours a day and we have an intuition that gives us invaluable information that only we have. I left this doctor's office knowing I would never allow myself to be restricted from participating in my own healthcare again, especially when it came to saving my life.

By viewing this from my perspective and not from my doctor's, I gave myself the support I needed. I wasn't about to allow this neurologist, or anyone else, to take from me what was mine and weaken me. Because of how I had been treated, I felt somewhat guarded when I went to my next appointment with the same neurologist the following week. Once seated and pleasantries were exchanged, he said he had bad news.

What could be worse than being told I'm going to die, I thought, staring at him in disbelief.

He said there was a 20 to 30 percent chance that I could also have a life-threatening condition called von Hippel Lindau disease. I was to see "a very gifted ophthalmologist as soon as possible."

This eye doctor specialized in treating eye diseases, and yet his waiting room was the most crowded one I'd ever seen. I wasn't sure what to make of this. I got tired of reading *People* and *Time* magazine, so I wasn't in the best mood when, after waiting for over an hour, I finally got to see this "gifted" doctor.

He was tall and thin, in his late fifties, and had short salt-and-pepper hair. His way of greeting me was to stare at my chest with a stupid smirk on his face. After sitting and positioning his stool uncomfortably close to my knees, he explained von Hippel Lindau disease.

Von Hippel was an eye doctor, and Lindau was a neurologist. Hemangioblastomas, the type of tumor I was diagnosed as having, were often found in the eyes, spine, and brain, which is what originally brought these two doctors together.

"Did your neurologist tell you von Hippel Lindau disease is life-threatening? This is why you need to be tested right away."

After giving me a thorough eye examination, an MRI was scheduled to look at my spine for additional tumors. Thankfully, none were found, so I was back to only worrying about the brain tumor.

Gary had wanted to come with me the first time I had an MRI test the week before. I booked the last appointment of the day so it wouldn't interfere with his work any more than necessary. Once there, I changed into a cotton white gown and was instructed not to move while the pictures were being taken.

"You'll know this is happening when you hear the machine make a soft thumping sound," a young female technician said. I was given headphones with a microphone attached so I could hear and talk with the technician when needed and listen to music to help pass the time.

In the days leading up to this, I was told that death would come soon. Naturally, I became anxious once inside this coffin-shaped machine. Like ravenous mosquitoes, my fears came inside with me. I'd been told MRIs make "a soft thumping sound" when taking pictures, but it was more like a loud, jarring jackhammer sound, which added to my nervousness.

This test took place during the time when MRIs first became available. Only one was available in D.C. and one in the suburbs. People were still learning to use them. After more than an hour had passed, "Oh Little Town of Bethlehem" abruptly halted in my ears and an apologetic-sounding female voice said they had technical problems and had to restart the test.

"Do you need to come out or are you okay?" she asked.

I didn't want Gary to wait any longer than necessary. And if I came out, I probably wouldn't be able to go back in.

"I'm okay," I said, telling myself I had to be.

"O Christmas Tree" began to play. I sang carol after carol in a soft, quivering voice, making up lyrics I didn't know. If I stopped singing, I was afraid I would cry. To give myself the courage I needed, I sang with more enthusiasm.

I was annoyed at myself for not knowing more lyrics when a disheartening thought occurred to me. *Would I ever get the chance to learn them? Would this be my last Christmas?*

Until I felt a cool sensation from tears pooling inside one ear, I didn't know I had been crying. Because the tears moved down my cheeks and I had been told not to move, I was afraid they would have to start the test again. I waited for "the voice" to scold me as my heart pounded, but the only thing I heard was another Christmas carol.

To celebrate my narrow escape, I sang a boisterous "Rockin' around the Christmas tree" until I gasped and fell silent. The microphone was by my mouth and the technician must have heard me singing!

I grew hot from embarrassment until my next thought made me smile.

I've been stuck inside this narrow plastic coffin for God only knows how long, through no fault of my own. I had a paid and captured audience, so why not have some fun with this?

With gusto I sang song after song, making up lyrics I didn't know while mimicking Billie Holiday, Ethel Merman, Bob Dylan, and more. Because my singing was bringing me comfort and helping pass the time, I really got into this by embellishing each carol with a *cha-cha-cha!* and *yeah, baby, baby!*

I had been stuck inside this torture chamber for almost three hours when the technician interrupted my free concert with an abrupt, "We're done now."

The bed beneath me moved, freeing me from my confining cell. I waited for the technician to come and release me. I waited and waited, but no one came, so I found my way back to the dressing room. Once I changed back into my street clothes, I stepped into the hallway, but it was pitch dark. I couldn't see a thing, and no one answered when I hollered hello.

With my right hand on the wall for guidance, I went looking for Gary. Walking slowly and carefully, after what seemed like an eternity, my hand bumped into a small sign. I leaned towards the wall until my nose almost touched it. The sign read, "Waiting Room."

I opened the door beside it and took tentative steps inside. A floor-to-ceiling glass window dominated the far side of the room. Lights from a high-rise building across the street created abstract shapes of diffused light over the floor and walls.

I could just barely see that metal chairs lined the room's perimeter. I scanned each one until I found Gary sitting kitty-corner across the room from where I stood. His head was lowered to his chest, cradled in his hands. Being only 5'6" and with his body slumped over, he looked like someone's forgotten, frightened child.

He popped up his head when I called his name, and squinted in my direction. I studied him and he studied me as I slowly walked towards him. I saw tears in his eyes and dark spots on the front of his light blue shirt. Only after I called his name a second time did he jump to his feet and run to me.

Hugging me so tightly it hurt, he said, "I thought you died. I didn't know what to do or where to go."

"I'm fine, Gary. Just shaken by how long the test took."

"I couldn't go home to an empty apartment. I didn't know who to call to claim your body. Oh God, Sandi. I thought you were dead. That you died while they were testing you."

"I'm sorry no one told you they had problems with the machine."

"I thought they'd find me here in the morning because I didn't know where else to go."

"No one told you they had to restart the test all over? I've been stuck inside the machine all this time. And everyone just went home and left us here?"

"I need to get home right away," Gary said.

I felt awful that no one had told him about the delay, but I was relieved to see him so happy that I hadn't died. Ever since being diagnosed, I wondered why he never said anything like, "You can always count on me," or, "I'll always be here for you," or why he hadn't tried to comfort me at all. At least now I had proof that he wasn't going to run the first chance he got.

While I felt bad for him, how he acted before my diagnosis was challenging enough. He had been draining me then, but now, with his anxiety intensified, he was wearing me out even more. After he convinced himself that I had died, he responded to his false beliefs and created more problems for both of us, as was his pattern.

Because of how he acted at the clinic after I told him I had a brain tumor, he apparently didn't learn from his inappropriate behavior. When we got home from this appointment, I offered to help him better cope with his emotions, but he only got angry at me.

***

I got additional opinions from neurologists who friends recommended.

"Because of the location of your tumor, in the center of your head and at the top of the brain stem, we can't even do a biopsy without doing more harm than good. The only way we'll know if your tumor is malignant or not is if cancer is found in other parts of your body or, to be blunt, you die."

Maybe not knowing is a good thing. This way, I can choose to believe it's benign.

"I'm sorry, Ms. Gold, but after reading your test results, there's nothing I can do for you either. My best guess is that you have about six months to a year to live."

All these doctors believe they know what every person's body is capable of doing? I'm going to have to prove them wrong.

"Sandra, I don't see how I can help you. If I were you, I would get my things in order."

My things? This neurologist thinks I'm sitting here caring about my things? No. This is his awkward way of saying I'm going to die.

"No, Ms. Gold. Quite frankly, just as the other doctors have told you, there's nothing I can do for you either. Because of the tumor's location, I wouldn't touch you with a ten-foot pole."

Me thinks this doctor's bedside manner could use some improvement.

"We only know your tumor is fast-growing. To answer your question, I can't tell you if it will be the size of a ping-pong ball, softball, or basketball next week. We have no way of knowing."

I hope they have painkillers strong enough if my head splits open and I get a splitting headache. Under different circumstances, this silly pun would be funny.

Looking back at my younger self in response to these doctors' foretelling words, I refused to allow my emotions to devour me. I was learning from Gary how *not* to act. I had also learned from my mother when I was young how overreacting emotionally only made things worse. I refused to say to Gary or anyone, "Help! I don't want to die!" and make things even more difficult for him, although Gary thought nothing of expressing his fears in front of me.

I never even cried when each doctor told me I would die. I only cried in front of Dr. Lynn Brallier, a counselor for the terminally ill I had begun seeing once a week. I'm not saying that stuffing my emotions inside me was a healthy thing. Today I know it isn't.

It didn't feel safe to cry in front of Gary. I cried alone in the shower instead. Even there, I protected myself from feeling my tears as they merged with the warm water streaming down my face.

I had never felt comfortable imposing my problems on anyone. I had avoided doing this since I was a child. Now I was upsetting everyone, which was one of the most difficult things about my diagnosis. It was especially difficult to see how upset Gary and my mother were, two people I had tried to protect long before I got sick.

Gary faithfully went to all of my appointments. With his photographic memory, he could repeat everything my doctors said. He volunteered to be my spokesperson and answered everyone's questions. He handled all of my insurance claims, which was a huge help.

I appreciated all that he was doing, but he was so theatrical, while I was striving to be grounded. Every time I attempted to discuss his behavior with him, he would explode in anger and make no attempt to understand how he was compromising both of us.

Weeks after my diagnosis, reality struck. On a cold January afternoon, I felt my ability to remain strong was slipping. I was home alone and feeling the weight of my problems and my sorrow. I thought about what I had accomplished in my 33 years of life. I was ashamed of myself for not achieving as much as my friends. What helped me was my art, of all things.

I thought about the paintings I'd done the past year: I'd painted a vase of dead pink carnations. And I painted a large dead fish hanging by its tail from a rope. I also drew a pencil sketch of a woman hugging a gravestone and I'd painted a monochromatic portrait of my father's mother who died from a brain tumor before I was born.

What?! Death has been following me all this time! Fear tore through me like a piercing arrow. I could hardly breathe. My death has just been confirmed. *I really am going to die.*

Wile E. Coyote, an old cartoon character, was forever realizing, as he hung precariously in the air, that he had just run off a cliff. Once he realized his dangerous predicament, he pedaled his skinny legs furiously to keep himself from falling. When death appeared in my paintings, I backpedaled, too, by taking long, slow, deep breaths in an attempt to calm myself.

How could I not have noticed this theme of death in my paintings before? Searching for answers and finding none, I redirected my attention: Would I rather follow the prognosis of five neurologists who think I will die or follow what's coming through my art?

Well, that's a no-brainer, I thought and laughed at my stupid pun.

The entire room sharpened and grew bright: The wooden coffee table in front of me and everything on it, the old gray television set across the room, the beige overstuffed chair to my left, suddenly seemed to glisten as I sat feeling bewildered.

Everything surrounding me had become crystal clear, crisp, shiny, and gleaming. Everywhere I looked was beautiful. I could only sit in awe and wonder what was going on.

Buster, my brown tabby cat, came running into the room at lightning speed and leaped onto my lap. He lifted his head and looked at me as if to say, "You really have to grasp the significance of this."

I was totally mystified, but I'd also never felt so loved and supported.

I knew deep in my heart—whether I lived or died—no longer did I have to worry. God was watching over me, loving me in a way I never felt loved before.

And from Buster, pure love radiated. His coloring and markings looked astonishing. His green eyes were more gorgeous than I had ever seen them look, and his face looked exceptionally adorable and sweet.

I felt honored to be living with such a loving creature, and humbled and grateful that this overseeing God was contacting me and using my language, reaching out through my art to let me know I was not alone.

How many people have experienced anything like this? I asked myself, as scenes from the Bible flashed through my mind, stories of imperfect people receiving miracles, messages like this, that changed their lives. *God works in mysterious ways*, I thought, and only then understood what this saying really meant.

I didn't want to do anything that would break this spell. I wanted this love to last forever. Remaining very still, I inhaled this feeling and thanked God for loving me in such a deep and significant way. As was my unhealthy habit, I questioned my worthiness, but caught myself by asking, *Who am I to question God?* and smiled at my absurdity.

My thoughts drifted to Gary, my family, and friends, wanting them and everyone to experience this kind of love. To retain this feeling of love fortifying and strengthening me for as long as I could, I chose to make love my guide until the day I died.

I had never heard the term Expressive Arts before, and I wouldn't for more than six more years. But on this January afternoon in 1987, I first understood how healing art was. From art I found my tether, my lifeline to life. Whether I lived or died, I wanted to attach myself to God's ankles and hang on tight. I wanted to live as close to Him as I possibly could. I decided the most effective way to do this was by following love, fully living my life, and being the person I was created to be.

For years, I never mentioned this to anyone. I couldn't afford to have people question it. I shared this love with others instead, especially with Gary, by supporting and reinforcing the help he was capable and willing to give. And I did my best to accept the ways that he couldn't.

I immediately signed up and took a class at the Smithsonian Institution on comparative religions. I sat in the audience in bliss, grateful to feel mankind's connectedness and our common need and desire to share our love with each other.

Each articulate speaker lovingly spoke about his religion. Every one had his own individual way of expressing the love and this connective adhesiveness within us all. Each of the speakers mesmerized me as they validated the love I felt and knew was going to save my life.

You'll Be Surprised How Strong You Are

I persevered until I got the appointment with Dr. Ojemann. I refused to be forced into a template by my neurologist where I knew I didn't fit. I felt proud my body was handling the tumor well. I knew I couldn't afford to worry about possibilities (such as possibly having von Hippel Lindau disease) because I had enough on my plate. To stop myself from getting overwhelmed, I sang in the MRI. I saw that Gary was in no shape to think of anything but his fears and didn't try to get him to understand my own frightening experience. I knew it wasn't safe to cry in front of him and only cried in the shower. And I embraced the love that I was given.

Write down the ways you have surprised yourself by acting strong.

_____

_____

_____

_____

_____

_____

Write down the times you didn't act as strong as you wished and you shamed yourself for this. In what ways in the future might you treat yourself with love and compassion instead?

_____

_____

_____

_____

_____

_____

5

Finding the Right Doctors for Yourself

Towards the end of January, Gary and I flew to Boston to meet Dr. Ojemann. This doctor's office was typical of Massachusetts General Hospital. Its dark wooden walls, dim lighting, and peculiar shape made it obvious the room had not been designed to be an office.

My mother and stepfather drove up from Connecticut to meet us and joined us in this cramped space behind Gary and me.

Not long after we were all seated, the doctor said something that floored me.

"This tumor will most likely cause your death, but no one can say for sure when. Even if you were to do nothing, which is what I suggest, you could, for example, lose your ability to feel."

"My ability to feel? What do you mean by this, doctor?"

"Imagine reaching into your pocket. In it is a handful of change, but because of the damage the tumor has done, you wouldn't be able to feel anything."

"Nothing?"

"You could also lose your eyesight, your hearing, and your ability to speak and move your legs and your arms. Your body could be affected in any number of ways."

I could feel myself grow hot as I squirmed in my seat.

"We have no way of knowing how your body might react, only that having a tumor in the pons is the worst place to have one because the pons affects so many of the body's functions."

I turned in my chair to check on my mother. Her face had turned a bright shade of red and her facial muscles had tightened to such an extent that my beautiful mother looked grotesque. Her husband's face, in contrast, was a ghostly white. I was afraid one of them might have a stroke. I asked Dr. Ojemann about the physician Dr. Horowitz thought might be able to help me.

He replied that this was indeed another option, though he wouldn't necessarily recommend it. When I pushed ahead by expressing my interest, he asked his assistant to call the physician Dr. Horowitz had suggested.

To my delight, this doctor, named Kjellberg (pronounced *chell-berg*), offered to see us right away. To put an end to this meeting and encourage my parents to drive back home, I jumped to my feet and turned around and thanked them both for coming. The look of relief on their faces confirmed my suspicions: they wanted to get out of there just as much as I wanted them to leave.

Dr. Raymond Kjellberg was using proton beam radiation to treat inoperable tumors in an unusual way. And he was the only doctor in the world who offered what he did. He had pioneered the use of the cyclotron machine for medical purposes, opening doors in the medical world and changing it forever. The cyclotron machine was used during World War II as a weapon, but Dr. Kjellberg used it every Tuesday to save the lives of seven patients who traveled to Boston from all around the world every week.

He greeted Gary and me warmly and explained how his treatment worked. He was a large man, over six feet tall, and must have weighed close to 300 pounds. He wasn't fat, just big all over. He had a huge head, hands, and feet, chestnut-colored hair, and freckly pink skin.

Knowing this man would save my life, I couldn't help but study him as he explained the procedure as if this was the first time he had described it to anyone. It surprised me that I would have to wait two years before I knew if it worked, and I silently laughed at myself. What did it matter how long it took if it saved my life?

I wondered as I sat before him how it must feel seeing patients no other doctor in the world could help. His sparkling amber eyes and mischievous grin revealed the fun that he was having. I watched him act like a little kid who knew he had something that I wanted. We both seemed to understand this inside joke and grinned at one another. I knew within moments of meeting him, if he accepted me as his patient, I would place my life in his hands. As if his time wasn't precious, when he finished talking, he asked if I had any questions.

I jumped at this chance to tell him how upsetting it was that I had developed a temper in the last few months. And how guilty and horrible I felt to suddenly have no control and to be yelling at Gary. I asked if this was from the brain tumor, and prayed that it was.

Taking his time to respond, he smiled as if he knew how much I yearned to hear his answer. Finally he said, "Five years ago, I would have told you that you were a spoiled brat."

Turning his bear-like body in his worn desk chair, he pointed his enormous paw of a hand towards his office entrance. "But so many people have walked through that door and told me the exact same thing you did, so I have to say yes. Your temper is most definitely a side-effect from the brain tumor."

I melted in my chair with relief, but kept my eyes glued on him, seeing that he had more to say.

Staring down at the dark wooden floor, he again took his time before he answered. He slowly raised his head, looked me in the eyes and chuckled. "Not a very pleasant one, is it?"

I laughed too at his sick joke because he was the first person who understood how horrible it was having a temper that wasn't my fault. I beamed with delight and appreciation.

Now I had the proof I needed! I had been telling Gary I thought the tumor had caused the temper issue ever since I was first diagnosed, but he still tormented me until my temper blew. He knew how scared and awful I felt every time I lost control. Now that he knew this wasn't my fault, I thought for sure he would want to protect me from this insufferable terror. Terror that I'd been experiencing for months while I felt like I was losing my mind.

"Wow! I bet we won't meet many people as accomplished and intelligent in both our lifetimes," Gary said as we walked towards the elevator. "I feel like we just reached Mount Sinai and were given a precious gift." I was glad he trusted Dr. Kjellberg as much I did, because this meant he had to believe what he said about the tumor causing the temper. Now we would enjoy our lives and live in peace.

***

"According to my tumor board, three out of five of the doctors think what you have looks more like an arteriovenous malformation, which is not a tumor at all," Dr. Kjellberg told me on the phone, about a week later.

"Really? That's good news, right?"

"An AVM is an abnormal collection of blood vessels."

He went on to explain that the problem was that these weakened vessels could erupt at any time. It usually happened when a person was in his thirties or when a woman gave birth.

"You're 33 and childless. Good thing you've never had a baby. I strongly advise against it."

My stomach turned.

"In most patients, when an AVM erupts, they experience a severe headache. But because yours is in the pons, if it erupts and bleeds, you'll be dead in about five seconds."

"Dying in seconds sounds good to me. I've hated the thought of Gary or my family having to take care of me as my health deteriorated." My eyes watered and my throat tightened. I had to pause for a moment. "Living with something like a time bomb in my head I know won't be easy, but it's only for two years." It was dawning on me how hard this would be. Two years was a long time.

"I'm going to need a lot of support, so I'm going to ask everyone to be extra nice to me. To not upset me in any way. Once people understand that stress can lead to my death, everyone has to be nice to me, right?"

"You're right, Sandi!" the doctor said while laughing. "You'll be helping others become kinder people. That's good. That's really good. I've never looked at it like this, nor have any of my patients that I know of. I'm going to suggest this to everyone from now on."

"We'll both be making the whole world a kinder place," I said.

"To be honest, it's hard for us to know exactly what you have because the pons is so compact that anything in there is hard to read."

Every doctor keeps referring to additional problems the pons causes.

"I think it's important that you call it whatever you're most comfortable with, an AVM or a brain tumor. No one can dispute whatever you choose, and the treatment is the same either way if you decide to use Proton Beam Radiation."

I've already decided. There is no doubt in my mind.

"I do need to tell you that, if indeed what's in your head is an AVM, there's a small chance that the treatment itself could cause it to bleed. This could cause your death. You have a tough decision to make."

But it feels like this is the right thing to do.

"We've been doing this procedure for almost 20 years, so we've had a lot of experience."

Twenty years? Then why didn't any of the neurologists know about this? Thankfully, Dr. Horowitz did.

"Oh, and another thing I must tell you: The pons is the area that's most likely to get radiation damage, but I believe the chances are slim. Radiation damage only occurs in the first two years following your treatment, so if you don't get it then, you won't get it."

Legally, he probably has to tell me this ... but the chances are slim.

"Whether you have an AVM or a brain tumor, we do have a long waiting list. Time is of the essence, so don't take too long deciding."

"I'm most comfortable calling it a brain tumor. Thank you for giving me this option and for thinking of my comfort." Touched by this man's sensitivity, I was having trouble talking, but I knew he deserved to know how much I appreciated what he was doing for me. "I also want to tell you that offering to help me this way after five neurologists said they could offer me nothing ... Words can't express how grateful I am. And yes, I would like to be on your waiting list, please."

This was the last conversation I had with this extraordinary man. I did see him when I returned for my treatment and we exchanged hellos, but he was busy doing something to save people's lives and I didn't want to interrupt him.

***

Days later, Gary told me that my mother was making things more difficult for him. "She keeps calling me and crying. Why isn't she calling your sister and why isn't your sister calling you? Your brother could at least write to you from Africa and offer his support. Your family is supposed to be supporting us, not the other way around."

I defended my family, annoyed that I had to explain that because they loved me, they were overwhelmed, but that when I needed them, they would help me in a heartbeat and make up for this lapsed time. I believed this with all my heart. The fact that most families rallied to support a sick family member right from the start was something I probably couldn't think about because it would have been too dangerous to face this reality in my vulnerable state.

Even after Gary pointed out that my family wasn't supporting me, I accepted how they acted, just as I had done all my life. He'd furrowed his brow in a questioning manner and looked at me like I had two heads. I looked at him like he just didn't get it, and hoped he would start supporting me in the way he thought that I deserved.

Shortly after, he thanked me for asking my mother to stop calling him and relieving him of this stress. But I hadn't. Perhaps my mother realized it wasn't healthy for her to be draining my main support system?

I understood why these calls stopped when I visited her, just a few months later. Her glassy eyes told me why she had changed. She appeared like those drunken cartoon characters with bubbles around their heads to give them that topsy-turvy, out-of-it look. I couldn't connect with her like I had been hoping. She had built a wall around herself using medication, just as she often did during challenging times.

"If this is what my mother needs to do, then this is what she needs," I decided. I still wonder what would have happened if I had been honest and told her how frustrating it was that she used drugs when I needed her, and it hurt that she hadn't made herself available to me. I wonder if she would have been willing to stop.

Had I been too respectful of her right to choose for herself while I sacrificed my obvious needs? What would have happened if I had honored myself and not put my mother's needs before mine? If I hadn't acquiesced to her wishes like I was raised to do and had always done, how different would our lives have been, or would anything have changed at all?

Feel Your Feelings and Let Love Guide You

I felt a strong connection when I first met Dr. Kjellberg. My heart opened wide. When he confirmed the temper issues were caused by the tumor, I felt deep gratitude, which opened my heart even more. After he advised me against having children, I kept my focus on my goal of staying alive. My body was telling me to listen to this man. And my mother? Admittedly, my blind love for her temporarily led me astray, but I did learn from this.

Write down the times you felt love and gratitude and those feelings guided you in a beneficial way.

_____

_____

_____

_____

_____

_____

_____

_____

Write down the times you may have missed an opportunity to feel appreciation or love and acted against yourself. Remember that being temporarily angry is not necessarily a negative thing.

_____

_____

_____

_____

_____

_____

_____

6

You Can't Afford to be a Doormat and Treat Yourself Unlovingly

At the beginning of February, I was home alone watching *Days of Our Lives* or perhaps it was *As the World Turns*. I had never watched a soap opera before, and after this period in my life I never would again. I may have been following Gary's example, except I was using television to distract myself from feeling my feelings instead of using drugs. Dr. Kjellberg's office called to say that an appointment was available and I could go for treatment in a few days. But I declined.

"It just doesn't seem natural," I later told Lynn, my therapist.

"Did you drive yourself here today?" she asked.

"Yes."

"And you use a telephone. And you cook on a stove. So, you don't object to using machines to assist your life. I'm merely suggesting that you think about this. I'll respect whatever you decide."

Shortly after, Dr. Kjellberg's office called with another opening. I decided that I was now ready, and Gary and I flew to Boston.

***

Having my head drilled was the only difficult part of the procedure. I was sitting in a large open room with people walking about, when four men wearing white lab coats and using Black and Decker drills bored holes in my cheeks and the back of my head and fastened screws into my bones. Simultaneously, two other men shot needles into my ears before inserting brass-pointed objects into them. These metal objects and the four screws

37

were then attached to a thick metal halo that encircled my head. Wingnuts were attached and tightened. This halo would be added to the cyclotron machine just prior to my treatment.

This was all completed in seconds. With twelve hands working this rapidly (eight drilling holes into my head), I opened my eyes so wide that I gave myself a black eye—the first of Dr. Kjellberg's patients ever to do this.

The treatment itself took less than ten minutes. While I sat on a metal chair, the end of what looked like an elephant trunk was securely placed on one side of my head. After the cyclotron machine hummed for a few minutes, my chair was spun around, and the other side of my head received the same treatment.

I only spent one night in the hospital before I flew home to start my two-year wait. Evidence of my treatment (besides my self-inflicted shiner) was covered by a small round Band-Aid on each of my cheeks.

On the plane home, there was an energetic strawberry-blonde toddler standing on her mother's lap and facing backward towards me. To help her mother keep her entertained, I made funny faces while smiling at her.

Seeing my black eye and the two round circles on my cheeks, the little girl laughed and shouted, "Mommy! Mommy! There's a clown on the plane!"

***

Many months passed. Late one night, Gary and I were watching *Roseanne* on TV. During a commercial, I ran into the kitchen for a glass of water, tripped on the fringe of our new kitchen rug, and broke my toe. When I screamed in pain, Gary ran into the kitchen. "That must really hurt because you're not a crybaby," he said.

At 2:00 in the morning I couldn't stand the pain any longer, so we went to the hospital to get a painkiller. The Chief of the Emergency Room called me later that day and told me an intern had been on duty and hadn't realized that a tumor in my toe had caused it to break. Because the tumor could be malignant, I had to go back and have a biopsy.

After hanging up the phone, I thought: *Since they couldn't do a biopsy on the brain tumor, I'd been told that cancer, if it was malignant, would be found elsewhere. Please God, don't let it be.* Thankfully, the tumor in my toe was benign. Having two tumors within months of each other, from head to toe, was just a bizarre coincidence.

Much later, while on vacation, a severe pain shot through my left shoulder as I was body surfing. I passed out in the water and almost drowned. Because I had begun seeing double the week before and it had not quite been two years since I had my treatment, I suspected I might have radiation damage.

Dr. Kjellberg's office instructed me to have another MRI and see an eye specialist. I was also told that because I was so close to my two-year "finish line," these test results would show if my treatment was a success or not. Feeling overjoyed that I would soon know, this was all that I focused on.

While lying inside the MRI, knowing that I would soon be getting this long-awaited news, I was jazzed. I kept thinking about getting my life back, without so many doctors in my life. Once released from the MRI, I was surprised to see a young radiologist standing by my feet.

"Hello, doctor," I said, smiling, thrilled my new life was about to begin.

"I can't find a problem in your head," he said.

I laughed and replied, "That's great news! I've been waiting to hear that for almost two years," to which he barked, "It's not good news until I say it's good news. I'm pumping you full of dye and having more pictures taken because I'm getting to the bottom of this!"

The only thing that mattered was Dr. Kjellberg's opinion, so I ignored his little hissy fit and focused on knowing that in just days, I would find out if the procedure was a success. I would have my freedom back—and my life.

***

I called Dr. Kjellberg's office every day, anxious to know my test results, but for some unknown reason, he never received my pictures. Growing more frustrated as each day passed, I called the hospital and was connected to this same unpleasant radiologist.

"Your doctor hasn't received your pictures because I haven't mailed them. I've been looking at them and—"

"What? *You've* been looking at them?"

"I never sent them because I think—"

"I've been calling Dr. Kjellberg's office every day, anxious to hear *his* opinion, not yours."

"The pictures showed—"

"Did you not hear me? What the f%@# is wrong with your brain?!

Silence followed before he replied, "Give me the address."

"You've proven you can't be trusted, so I'm going to come and get them and mail them myself," I said before I slammed down the phone.

I called my mother to update her and confessed what I said to this doctor.

"Good for you, Sandi. Give 'em hell!" I was happy to hear her say.

I called Gary to tell him why Dr. Kjellberg's office hadn't gotten my pictures since he, too, had been wondering why there was this long delay. He kindly offered to pick them up and have his secretary mail them.

"Thank you so much," I said to him when he got home. "I assume you didn't see that egotistical radiologist."

"In fact, I did. His name is Dr. Lewis, and he's a nice guy. We had a good laugh over how hysterical menstruating women can be."

I was already aware of his pattern. Quintessential of an addict's behavior, Gary would attempt to aggravate me when he knew I was particularly vulnerable. Whenever he had a need to create drama he'd provoke a fight.

I remained silent and just stared at him while thinking, *Is he so emotionally damaged that he really just stooped this low?*

***

I waited for over an hour in the waiting room for my second appointment with this same ophthalmologist who had kept me waiting before. Between this guy and the radiologist, I was tired of their misplaced sense of entitlement. When my name was finally called, I was escorted to the examination room and had to wait another ten minutes before the doctor strolled in.

Once he was seated, he aggressively wheeled his stool in front of me and leaned his face close to mine and said, "Don't you ever speak to any doctor the way you spoke to Dr. Lewis."

Instinctively, my spine straightened as my body pulled away. Less than two feet from me, a light bulb exploded in a green goose-neck desk lamp, making a loud gunshot sound. The doctor jumped to his feet and looked at me with a look of fear and confusion. Calmly, I gave him my best Mona Lisa smile to add to his discomfort. He moved his head back and forth from the lamp to me before he scurried from the room. Five minutes later, he returned with a smug look on his face and took his position on his stool again.

"Like it or not, you're having another MRI, young lady," he said, while writing something down to record this.

Like hell I am, I thought.

In the upper right-hand corner of the room, a deep-dish stainless-steel pan crashed onto the floor with a loud metallic vibrating sound. The doctor jumped to his feet again and wrapped his arms around his thin body, looking like he was about to cry.

I'm in control of my own healthcare even if you, Dr. Lewis, or anyone else tries to take this from me.

"Are you all right?" the doctor asked.

"Are *you*?" I answered, looking at him in a way that suggested he had better not mess with me again. I hadn't known I was capable of doing psychokinesis, but I now believe if we are pushed too far, our ability to protect ourselves can become intensified, just as mine did.

"Please make sure the results of this examination are promptly sent to Dr. Raymond Kjellberg at the Massachusetts General Hospital, who's overseeing my health care. I've already left his address at the front desk," I purposely said in a haughty manner before I sweetly smiled.

I fought to keep myself from giggling as I stood and left this bewildered man who still had his arms wrapped around himself.

Dr. Kjellberg got the test results he requested. Shortly afterward, I received a letter from him congratulating me on my success. After waiting almost two years and overcoming many obstacles, no sign of radiation damage was found, and my life was no longer threatened.

Know Your Priorities

I waited and had the treatment when it felt right to me, after I did what I needed to do to prepare myself. I rolled with the punches: no broken toe, shoulder pain and almost drowning, an obnoxious eye doctor, Gary's behavior, or a controlling radiologist had defeated me. I kept my focus on reaching my goal.

Write down the times you set priorities and you let nothing get in the way of obtaining them.

_____

_____

_____

_____

_____

_____

_____

_____

Write down the times you set priorities, but you became distracted and defeated, and why. What might you have done better to reach your goal? What did this cost you?

_____

_____

_____

_____

_____

_____

_____

_____

7

Identify What You Are Responsible for and What is the Responsibility of Others

It's common for someone to think marijuana only causes psychological dependence. I believed this too, before I lived with Gary. Having a life-threatening brain tumor wasn't easy, but living with the repercussions of Gary's addiction made this even more difficult. Because I was feeling particularly stressed, I attended my first 12-step meeting just before I learned the treatment had been successful.

It was in 1989 when I started going to ACOA meetings (for Adult Children of Alcoholics), Al-Anon meetings (for people who love an addict), and CODA meetings (for people who share a common desire to develop functional and healthy relationships) several times a week.

Days after I received Dr. Kjellberg's congratulatory letter, I was relaxing in the living room and reading *Recovery: A Guide for Adult Children of Alcoholics*.

Silently, Gary walked over to me, encircled his arms tightly around my shoulders, and buried his face in my long hair. He said I was the kindest person he'd ever met, but also that he was leaving me. *Why hadn't he ever told me he thought I was this kind before?*

With his arms still clasped around me (to avoid eye contact?) I asked why he had never been willing to talk about his unhappiness to give us a chance at resolving our problems.

As if I had thrown acid in his face, he released his grip, jumped back, and shouted, "You're a sensitive person, Sandi. You should have known I wasn't happy. I shouldn't have to tell you."

He believed my job was to figure out what he wanted as if we were playing a game of charades? Because he didn't have the courage to speak his truth, he had been screaming at me in frustration for years, expecting me to understand him in a language that was foreign to me. Because he refused to take responsibility for himself, he put this responsibility on me. It was the typical behavior of a drug addict.

The week before, for the first time, he had attempted to stop smoking dope. He was shocked and badly shaken when he discovered he could only go three days before he had to smoke again. Since he could no longer deny he was addicted, rather than apologize for the hell he put me through, he became livid with me.

I had no idea he'd been trying to stop. After I promised Pamela I would never talk about it, I taught myself to ignore his smoking. Even after Gary refused to continue going to counseling, I never said anything about his drug habit.

Believing he had a right to make this decision as Pamela had taught me, and that this was the most loving and respectful thing I could do for him, I left this responsibility to Gary, which apparently, he didn't appreciate.

After I was diagnosed with the brain tumor, I thought for sure he would have wanted to make my life easier. I waited for him to stop smoking while never saying anything about this. Eventually, I gave up hoping and just ignored it.

While he was lying on the couch the week before, I innocently asked what the foul smell was. His head snapped up and his eyes popped open before he ran from the room. This was how I realized that he had stopped smoking, and what I smelled was the putrid stench from his body purging 15 years of accumulating toxins.

Still, I respected his privacy and never said anything about this to him or anyone. And yet every time he saw me in the days that followed, he glared at me in anger like a pissed-off teenager. I had no desire to engage with this, so I just ignored it.

For years, I had waited for Gary to realize that he, I, and our relationship deserved so much more than he was willing to give. But his addiction, and his need to avoid responsibility, apparently took precedence.

***

I moved back to New England, close to Groton Long Point, where I grew up, supported by the expansive sea and nature's beauty all along the scenic coast that provided me with the unlimited spaciousness and peace that I needed. I rented a studio in Westerly, Rhode Island, where I painted almost every day. I lived on a friend's sailboat in the picturesque Stonington harbor, moored just a stone's throw away from a navy blue-hulled sailboat owned by Christopher Reeve.

As the sun rose each morning, I would sit on the deck and thank God for my life. I slept like a baby, rocked to sleep by the gentle waves every night. I could not have found a better way to heal from my unhealthy relationship with Gary and the hell from the brain tumor. I felt profound gratitude that I had landed on a boat with a million-dollar view, greeted by white swans each morning. I loved sitting on the bow and inhaling the fresh salt air while enjoying the warmth of the rising sun. My plan had been to leave my health problems back in D.C. and give myself the freedom to live my life without this heavy baggage. But I kept feeling a persistent need to let others know about Dr. Kjellberg's little-known treatment that could save other people's lives.

In 1992, two years after I returned to New England, I co-founded the Artist Cooperative of Westerly to form and ignite a local arts community in downtown Westerly. Webster Terhune was the curator of the Hoxie Gallery, the most gorgeous, but underutilized gallery in the area. He walked down an alley and along the Pawcatuck River to get to my studio and see my art, and possibly offer me an art show. Before he arrived, to demonstrate I was still growing as an artist, I put my work in chronological order, something I had never done before or since.

As he viewed my art, I nervously held my breath until he pointed to one of my pieces and asked, "What happened here? Why does the artwork suddenly have an extraordinary, almost desperate intimacy to it? It's as if you painted it with another set of eyes, almost from the inside out."

I was so stunned I couldn't speak because he pointed to the first piece I'd painted after I was diagnosed with the brain tumor. A stimulating conversation about life, death, and art followed, with Webster asking me many questions. He suggested I paint a mural in his gallery to share what I had just told him.

"Only if I can erase it," I said and watched his jaw drop. "Because life is temporary, the mural has to be."

"You won't believe this, but I was thinking the same thing. You'd really be willing to paint something as large as a mural and then erase it?"

"Yes. For over two years I had to find ways to make peace with my possible death, which was like having to find a way to befriend a boa constrictor wrapped around my neck. I discovered using love was the only way, and this is what I plan to paint into the mural. I want people to feel this."

"I'm looking forward to seeing how you do this. Tell me more about how love and the brain tumor changed you. I'm really interested."

"I discovered I couldn't feel fear and appreciation simultaneously. That appreciation, making the most of every moment, loving life, and living in the present gave me strength."

"Please go on."

"Finding ways to feel grateful is what changed, defined, and reshaped me and my life."

"Can you give me specific examples?" Webster asked.

"By appreciating what we have, such as the joy we feel noticing a pink-cheeked baby staring lovingly into her mother's eyes, or the smell of freshly laundered sheets as we climb into bed. How we view everyday things can change our lives."

For years, I had thought about how I would express what I learned. And how to let people know about the treatment. Talking with Webster that first day I met him gave me the answer.

I had committed to painting something that people would have to care about when I erased it, putting a huge amount of pressure on myself.

***

In September 1993, I went to work on this project. It took me three months, painting seven days a week, to complete it.

As soon as I started, word quickly spread. The local newspapers and television programs reported on my progress at least once a week. After the Associated Press wrote an article about it and periodically sent updates that appeared in newspapers all throughout the United States, the media coverage exploded.

The ABC news show *20/20* came and took three days to film their segment. I was interviewed by Catherine Crier, an Emmy award-winning journalist, who impressed me by joining me and my friends for lunch and eating a hot chili pepper without flinching at all.

"I'm from Texas," she proudly proclaimed.

After Barbara Walters introduced my story to six million viewers, it became one of *20/20*'s top three most popular stories that year.

The Boston Globe, People Magazine, USA Today, The Providence Journal, The Rocky Mountain News, The Augusta Chronicle, The Phoenix Gazette, The Orlando Sentinel, and hundreds of other news outlets across the country published stories about the mural.

Susan Stamberg interviewed me on National Public Radio, and Faith Middleton on Connecticut Public Radio. Representatives from the Polaroid Corporation came. They told me they were sent by the owner of the company to help me in whatever way they could; that my story had touched him so much, he wanted "to help me become a millionaire."

I sincerely thanked them, and respectfully explained that I didn't paint the mural to make money. But to take advantage of this opportunity, I created the Gold/Kjellberg Foundation at Massachusetts General Hospital to help people who couldn't afford the treatment I had. *20/20* agreed to announce that viewers could donate to the foundation by buying a framed Polaroid print of the mural. Polaroid then took days meticulously photographing it, in the same way they photograph famous paintings in museums to replace those on loan.

Three times my story made the headlines in my hometown newspaper, *The Westerly Sun*. Photographers from all three local papers—*The Norwich Bulletin, The New London Day*, and *The Sun*—photographed me at least once a week for three months. Updates of my story were often broadcast on all three local news stations the same night.

Three months after the opening night, the mural had accomplished everything I hoped for, and more. I erased it as I'd planned. (The video of me erasing it can be seen on my website www.sandigold.com.) Even though decades have passed, I can still see the mural in my mind's eye. Below the blue watery horizon at the top, in a majestic and proud manner, I painted a large three-story temple, 63' wide and 15' high, that consisted of nearly 50 windows framed in brown and black. Inside these dark frames, I painted local scenes that had captured my attention during my walks. I'd felt as if each had been waving at me, beckoning for me to notice them, sort of winking at me to offer me their love and support.

By including these colorful glimpses of captivating beauty in various shaped windows that looked vaguely religious, I passed on the love that I had been given so others would feel it too. My intention was to encourage others to stop and allow their hearts to be touched in the same way that had helped save my life.

Most people walk by and lose these life-sustaining opportunities without realizing what they're missing, or the price they're paying by not noticing the love and beauty in these treasured moments. I wanted to show how these everyday experiences can permeate and strengthen our bodies, and improve our health and happiness.

An estimated 10,000 people came to see the mural during the 30 days it was on display. Many stood looking at it with tears in their eyes. One woman said she saw the mural as a thank you note to God. Another shared that she felt my love had touched her so deeply it was now inside her. One man, as he wiped his eyes with his handkerchief, spoke to me about his dying wife telling him about the love and appreciation she felt as she was dying. And that only now that he had seen the mural, did he understand what she was trying to tell him.

One of the most memorable reactions occurred when a couple from South Carolina drove non-stop up to Rhode Island to see the mural after the woman had a bone marrow transplant. They arrived at the library 15 minutes before closing and practically danced around the gallery, giggling like two small school children. Webster offered to keep the library open late so they could enjoy their experience further.

"Just seeing it. Just standing in front of it for 15 minutes and feeling the love the artist poured into it is more than enough for me," this appreciative woman exclaimed.

***

As an older, wiser me, now in my late sixties, I understand what Webster saw. My paintings changed because I changed. Because I learned to embrace the very things I used to shield myself from—my pain and vulnerability—powerful, life-changing shifts occurred.

I discovered that when we retreat in fear, hide, or live in bitterness and anger, when we try to pretend we're something that we're not, we harm ourselves and our lives. Every one of us was created with something to benefit the world, which is why it's imperative that we be true to ourselves.

Webster saw this change in my art. It wasn't until people began asking me questions, treating me like I had something that they wanted, something I could contribute to their lives, and that I was deserving of their respect, that I began to recognize the ways I had grown. I felt more seen and accepted for who I was.

Initially, I found people's interest in me puzzling, but gradually, as more people's curiosity grew, I began to understand why so many people were interested by me. At first, because it was new and strange, I didn't think I deserved all this attention and the compliments I got. It surprised me that so many people wanted to know my beliefs without being critical or imposing their beliefs on me. People no longer believed they knew what my personal experience should be or how I was supposed to act. This didn't mean every person treated me in a loving and respectful way, but those who acted differently drew attention to themselves like a flashing red neon sign.

Getting the Help You Need

Because I was at my wit's end, I began attending 12-step meetings where I learned I had to stop fixating on Gary's problems and work on myself. After I moved to New England, I wanted to find a way to let people know about Dr. Kjellberg's procedure. Once I started painting, I got a lot of help from the media. Word spread fast and my career began to surge. Because I had been true to myself, I got the help I needed to fulfill my goals.

Many people have a difficult time asking for help. They may even fool themselves into believing they don't need it. Write down the ways you've asked for help from others and how you benefited because you did.

_____

_____

_____

_____

_____

_____

Write down the times you didn't ask for help to your detriment, and what this cost you. In what ways might you have gotten help had you asked?

_____

_____

_____

_____

_____

_____

_____

8

Know Who's Got Your Back

Nine months after erasing the mural, I was sitting by my easel, concentrating on painting. I didn't hear my friend Gainor walk into the studio we shared.

"Why are you painting with your right hand when you're left-handed, San?"

Because my left hand had started cramping whenever I painted or wrote with it, I completed sections of the mural with my non-dominant right hand. There was no way I could accept I had more health problems, so I adapted. When Gainor asked me this question, I could only cry. I was scared I had radiation damage.

I had been ignoring these symptoms, problems not just with my hand, but with my eyes and balance. I still painted, but with my right hand. Since I continued to win awards, I must have told myself that all was well. The other thing that probably contributed to my denial is that I had no health insurance. I couldn't afford to be sick.

Using his skills as an attorney, almost ten years before, Gary had tried to fight my escalating health insurance premiums. But because D.C. wasn't a state, it had no insurance commissioner who could help.

Shortly after I moved to New England, my mother told me I was causing problems with her relationship with her mother, after my grandmother complained about paying the escalating costs of my health insurance. I didn't know what my mother expected me to do, since she knew I couldn't afford to pay for it. And yet, she kept bringing this subject up, unwilling to let it go. To stop this unhealthy stress that I couldn't afford to have, I dropped my health insurance and made every effort to live as healthfully as I could. I thought this was the most responsible thing I could do.

When symptoms from the radiation damage first appeared, I must have convinced myself that whatever was happening to my body would go away. Plus, Dr. Kjellberg had died of lung cancer just months before. His death probably contributed to my denial that I had problems, too.

"Don't cry, San. We don't have to tell anyone. We won't even tell your mother, because I know how irrational she gets. You have to think about yourself, as hard as I know this is for you," Gainor said.

"I know I have radiation damage. I don't have health insurance and I don't want to live in debt for the rest of my life."

"For God's sake, you opened a foundation at the hospital for people who need financial assistance. Well, you're now the one who needs it. Call your doctor. I'm sorry, but I'm not leaving until you do."

***

"I think I have radiation damage," I said to the doctor who had taken Dr. Kjellberg's place, as I sat before him with Gainor at my side. "My left hand cramps, and I'm left-handed. And my balance is off. I have to hold on to walls when I'm tired 'cause I lose my balance. I'm seeing double too, though this comes and goes."

"What you're saying is impossible, Ms. Gold."

Oh, brother. Here we go again.

I was told if I had radiation damage, it would have occurred within two years of my treatment. It had now been over seven. They had never had a patient get radiation damage after two years, so they falsely believed this was not possible. The doctor suggested they take some tests to "see what's really going on inside your head, but I can assure you that you don't have radiation damage."

A week later, I returned to the hospital for these test results with my mother, who had insisted on coming.

"This is a family matter. You can't take Gainor," she said. And in my wearied state, I acquiesced to her insistence that she come to support me instead of Gainor.

"Ms. Gold, after reviewing your tests, I'm sorry to have to tell you that you have radiation damage."

Are you kidding me? This doctor is pretending I hadn't just told him this?

"And because our tests are more sophisticated today than they were before, we can now see that a part of the AVM still remains. I can't tell you that it's no longer life-threatening, but there's nothing we can do about this, anyway."

"Noooooooooooooooooooooooooooooo! I'll sell my house! Don't let my daughter die! No. No. No," my mother yelled at the top of her lungs as she sobbed and flung her arms in the air.

I had just been told I could drop dead any moment for a second time in my life, after Dr. Kjellberg—my favorite doctor—had told me my life was no longer threatened. At the same time, I heard my mother screaming about my potential death and selling her home to save me. And Gainor wasn't there to support me.

Guilt hit me like a tidal wave. I'd broken our family rule—never upset Mom. If my mother lost her home, my siblings would brutally punish me. My mother screaming and falling apart, threatening to sell her house, and hearing that I had radiation damage, *and* the AVM was still in my brain and I could die in seconds again, was too much for me to digest. But no one was thinking about my emotional state. I ran to comfort my mother.

"And regretfully, Dr. Kjellberg donated all his records to a small hospital out west, so we don't have access to yours," I remember hearing, but the doctor's voice was fading because my body was shutting down.

Until my appointment the following week, I tortured myself with my thoughts, just like Gary used to do to me. I feared I would look like the victims of Hiroshima. I was told that the time bomb was in my head and could kill me in seconds again. In my discombobulated state, I must have combined these two bombs, or perhaps, intuitively, I knew a bomb was about to explode in my life.

While driving home from the hospital, since I was about to be heavily medicated for who knows how long, my mother suggested I move in with her. The two of us had always been close and got along well as long as I obeyed the family rule and didn't upset her. Her need for excitement had left me captivated as a child. Maybe it was because my siblings, in comparison, kept everything inside. I used to think of my mother as a goddess who electrified my life. I cherished our relationship, especially since neither of my siblings had a close relationship with her. Because I did, I felt special.

"I thought she was immature," my sister told me when we were young adults. "You were the baby, so it was different for you. I couldn't understand why she acted so irresponsibly when she was supposed to be the grown-up. Remember, there's always an element of truth to what she says, but you never can trust her."

The older I got, I was able to see how right my sister was. I wished I hadn't been so easy to fool and manipulate when I was young, as though a spell had been cast over me, making me blindly love and defend my mother. In hindsight, I wish she had been more mature and had understood that her children needed and deserved a mother who could offer us stability.

A few days after we returned from the hospital, my mother told me she had just seen a naturopathic physician who suggested she get a prescription for her anxiety. I replied that not having her available when she depended on medication after I got a brain tumor had been hard on me and that I'd felt guilty that she did.

"I never knew you knew," she said nervously, jerking her head.

"I didn't tell you because I didn't want to take this security from you, Mom."

Suspecting my mother was fibbing about what the naturopathic doctor told her, I said, "You went to him wanting a natural treatment—not a drug. I'm going to call and give him hell."

"No! Don't call his office. Maybe I misunderstood. Don't call on my behalf," my mother said, confirming my suspicion.

She was someone who never could speak her truth. Her insecurities irritated my siblings, but I'd always seen her behavior as a call for love. I told her that I needed her more than ever because having radiation damage terrified me; that together we would help one another get through this.

Because I was their first patient to get radiation damage more than two years after treatment, my case piqued my doctors' interest. Or maybe it was because I had created the Gold/Kjellberg Foundation that brought attention and lots of money to the hospital. Or maybe they thought they could learn from my case. Whatever the reason, three neurosurgeons volunteered their help, and the hospital waived its fee, so selling my mother's house was not necessary, much to my relief.

These three doctors decided to treat me using steroids even though "they weren't pleasant." But steroids proved to be far more than just unpleasant. They were depressants, and I became more depressed than I thought was possible. Until my body adjusted, I could hardly walk. I felt like I was falling down a deep and dark stone well and nasty, sharp-clawed creatures from inside the walls were reaching out, trying to tear me apart.

When I told my doctors how miserable I was, they gave me anti-depressants. Because the steroids kept me awake at night, they gave me sleeping pills, too. I had never even kept aspirin in my home before I got the brain tumor, so my body was highly susceptible to being medicated. And yet, even after taking this many drugs, I couldn't help seeing how petrified my mother was. Rather than protect me from knowing how scared she was, it was as if she wanted me to see her like this, just like Gary used to do.

It felt like I was being manipulated, as if my mother wanted me to feel guilty for "doing this" to her. This confused me because she knew how scared I was. And that I needed *her* support. I had never asked for any help in the seven years before this, since I was first diagnosed with the brain tumor. I had told my mother I was terrified by the radiation damage, so why was she looking at me as though I was some kind of monster?

***

When I was on steroids, I lost all sense of being connected to the world. I even lost my ability to pray, something I didn't know was possible to lose. When Buster, my cat, jumped onto my lap, and I felt nothing, no love for him, I knew I needed to get professional help.

Being told, just days before being given depressants, the AVM had never completely left my head and could kill me again in seconds, added to my anxiety. Every fear I had ever stifled since being diagnosed with the brain tumor took advantage of my medicated state and surfaced. I was an emotional wreck. And every time my mother looked at me in terror, I was overwhelmed by guilt.

This feeling of being manipulated by my mother must be a side effect of the steroids, I thought. "It's not as though I killed someone while driving drunk, or I had infected someone with AIDS, so why am I feeling like such a despicable person?" I asked my mother, but she only stared at me.

My mother was a petite, small-boned woman. She has always been emotionally frail. Ever since I was a child, she had leaned on me. She'd always told me that no one could understand and help her in the way that I could. Because I was made to feel like she needed me, and I had this ability that no one else had, I was always happy to help her.

While on steroids, in this medicated state, I couldn't give my mother the attention she relied on. Expecting my siblings to help her now, she called and complained to them about how cold and cruel I'd become. I had always tried to insulate my siblings from our mother's emotional needs, but I couldn't while I was on steroids. Having our mother lean on them proved to be overwhelming, just as it had been for Gary almost ten years before when she called him for his help.

Sadly, my brother and sister had learned their poor emotional skills from our mother, so they quickly became depleted. And just like her, their habitual reaction was to blame someone else for how they felt. It didn't take long before all three of them—bonded by their misery, fears, and anger—turned on me.

I was dumbfounded. And what made this particularly difficult was that none of them would explain what I had done that made them so angry. I had no idea why three people I had loved all my life were not helping me at my most vulnerable time, but had turned against me instead.

I tried to imagine how difficult it must be for a mother to see her daughter as sick as I was, especially since playing Florence Nightingale was not my mother's thing. I suspected that my siblings' desire to help her exceeded their emotional abilities, and they didn't know what else to do but demand that I help them. But it was impossible for me to help anyone in the state I was in, as hard as I was trying. The more my mother cried and expected my siblings to help her, the more frustrated and aggravated they became.

Before I got radiation damage, I had saved a gray flier from a Dr. Lori Leyden, who specialized in holistic stress management counseling. When my cat Buster jumped on my lap and I felt nothing for him, it was Lori who I called for help.

Denial is an Insidious and Costly Thing

Despite not being able to paint with my dominant hand, seeing double and losing my balance, I denied I had a problem. Just as I had done when I was young, I adapted. When I was told for a second time that I could die in five seconds and I had radiation damage, I denied I needed support. Instead, I comforted my mother. I also denied the effect my family's anger had on me for a long time. Because I did, the effect these traumas had on me lasted much longer.

Write down the times you were able to recognize that you had been in denial and you finally got help for yourself.

_____

_____

_____

_____

_____

_____

_____

_____

Write down the times you were in denial and didn't ask for the help you needed. In what ways did this cost you?

_____

_____

_____

_____

_____

_____

_____

_____

9

Find a Body-Centered Counselor Who Specializes in Traumas

"So, your mother is acting terrified. This mustn't be very comforting. It sounds like you could use some emotional support. Yes?" Lori said at our first appointment.

"She's doing all that she can for me. Cooking and doing my wash. She drove me here because I can't drive while on steroids, but she's always been emotionally fragile."

"From what I'm hearing you say, it sounds like your mother, your caretaker, can't give you comfort. That you've been trying your best to comfort her, but no matter how hard you try, you're not able. Is this true?"

"I've been doing all I can to comfort my mother my entire life, but now, because I'm medicated, I can't. Her fears have now turned to anger. It feels like she blames me for abandoning her just because I got sick."

"It appears as if you're focusing only on your mother, which shows that you have a huge heart, even under these circumstances. But your focus needs to be on you to help yourself get well. Doesn't this make sense? You made your health problems sound like a walk in the park compared to your mother's problems, and this concerns me."

"But my mother is falling apart because I got sick."

"You are only responsible for yourself. Your mother is an adult, and you are not responsible for her, even if she and your siblings expect you to be. I can see how upset you are. I'm going to give you some guided meditation tapes to listen to if you'd like."

"Tapes? What will they do?"

"They'll help to balance your nervous system. I suggest listening to them, alone in your room, several times a day. Once your body feels safe, this will support your immune system. Safety is the key to getting well."

"Thank you, Lori. I'll listen to the tapes all day if they'll help. Do you think my mother would benefit from listening to them, too?"

From Lori, I learned I had to focus on myself and my own healing if I wanted to get well. I had to stop being an enabler and stop playing the sacrificial lamb, putting everyone's needs before my own. Lori was the first person to encourage me to listen to my body for answers "because our bodies never lie, and are always trying to help us."

My mother showed no interest in listening to the tapes to help calm her anxiety. I realized she was doing nothing to help herself relax. Instead, she would manipulate and use guilt to get me and my siblings to help her.

It was during this time that I recognized I had been spending way too much time assisting and protecting her all my life. For both our sakes, I had to change, but whenever I complimented her on how well she did something, she seemed to resent it.

I had thought my mother appreciated that I overcame death years before without asking her for help. Even though no one in my family ever complimented me for what I'd achieved, never told me they were glad I lived or that I made them proud, I just assumed my family recognized and was grateful for my abilities and independence.

Lori taught me to never assume people were how I wanted and expected them to be; that not everyone lives from their heart, as I thought the members of my family did.

I had been living under the false impression that since my track record left no doubt of my competence, my family would respect whatever choices I made. But all three of them thought they knew better. They all kept telling me what to do, and kept getting angry at me because I chose to follow my heart.

In the mid-1980s, just before being diagnosed with the brain tumor, I was volunteering at the Torpedo Factory's Cooperative Gallery in Alexandria, Virginia, about 20 minutes from my home in Washington, D. C. While I was manning the front desk, a woman in her forties with short dark hair walked in and turned her back on me. When I saw that she was crying, I realized she had entered the gallery to compose herself. Slowly, I approached her, handed her a tissue, and asked if I could help. She told me she had cancer.

"But the cancer isn't the reason I'm crying. The worst part is how relatives I've loved my entire life act like I did something to them," she explained between sobs. "People I love, and I thought loved me, are being so cruel to me now. Some are even dropping out of my life." I couldn't imagine anyone treating someone like this. I told myself that having cancer had to be overwhelming her, but today I understand, more than I wish I did.

What made my family turning against me particularly difficult was that they still looked like they always did. But after I got radiation damage, they reminded me of the zombies in *The Night of the Living Dead*, creatures who could only think about getting their own needs met and would go to any length to do so, even if it threatened my life.

It's Important You Know You Are Worthy

From Lori, I learned I had to focus on myself if I wanted to get well, stop being an enabler and a sacrificial lamb, and putting others' needs before my own. Lori encouraged me to listen to my body for answers. From her, I learned that our bodies never lie, and I should not assume people were how I wanted and expected them to be; that not everyone lives from their heart. She applauded my choice to use love as my guide and encouraged me to follow my heart, influencing my ability to heal using love.

Many people have a difficult time accepting that they are worthy. Every morning, before you brush your teeth, look at yourself in the mirror, smile at yourself and say, "I love you." (I still do this.)

Write down the ways you acted against yourself, and acquiesced to others' needs and desires to your own detriment. What was the outcome because you did? And what did this cost you?

_____

_____

_____

_____

_____

_____

_____

_____

_____

_____

_____

_____

_____

10

You Can't Always Trust Your Doctors

After a year on steroids, this medication accomplished nothing. Zero. Zilch. I was disappointed and frustrated, to say the least. Another medication called Trental was then prescribed.

My doctors said it had no side effects. It would make my red blood cells more flexible, so they could reshape themselves and slip into the area of my brain that was damaged, bringing oxygen in to heal it. It took a month to make a new red blood cells so more patience was asked of me.

Getting off the steroids gave me more independence. I embraced my new freedom by taking long walks around my home in Groton Long Point. Frequently, I would stop and sit on East Dock or stand along the highest ridge that had water far below it, open my arms wide at shoulder level and close my eyes and face the Long Island Sound.

I used the massive expanse of water and the soothing sounds of the water splashing against the seaweed and barnacle-covered rocks below to nurture and comfort me. I'd deeply inhale the fresh salt air to strengthen my wearied spirit and imagined this energy healing my body.

I walked for miles every day, grateful for every step I took until, as the weeks turned into months, an unwelcome sensation accompanied me. I tried to convince myself that nothing was wrong, but I couldn't deny I was weakening. *Was the radiation damage now spreading to my organs? Was I slowly dying?*

These precious daily walks were hampered by a feeling that the light inside me was dimming. I wasn't getting better on this second medication. I was getting worse. Until I could process this, knowing my mother's angry reaction would only make things more difficult for me, I kept to my everyday walking schedule, but instead of completing my daily walk, I'd sit alone on South Beach. As a cool wind blew, I prayed and thanked God for watching over me until I felt it was safe to go home.

At my next appointment in Boston, I told my doctors I felt like something inside me was dying.

"What? According to all the tests we've taken, you're doing measurably better," they said, meaning how I tested was more important? "You probably just need rest from all the changes to your body." Not one question was asked of me. Since my doctors were reaching their goals, they showed no interest in hearing my perspective.

After investing almost two years of my life doing everything that was asked of me, my faith in my doctors vanished. I began having panic attacks. I thought I was having seizures until Lori asked, "Have you been feeling your feelings? My experience has shown if we ignore them, they're going to find ways to get our attention in unwelcomed, and often unpleasant ways. I think you're having panic attacks. Your body needs your attention."

"I thought I was feeling my feelings, though all this stress may be distracting me."

"As I see it, and tell me if you think I'm wrong, you don't feel safe in your home and it's even worse when your siblings visit. You don't feel safe in your doctors' hands, and you aren't getting better. I think how your body is responding makes perfect sense. Do you agree?"

Pausing for a moment, Lori's intense blue eyes studied me. "Could it be that your body feels ignored? I suggest feeling whatever you're feeling, no matter how frightening this may be."

"But I *have* been, Lori ... or I thought I was."

"Is it possible that you're afraid to tell your doctors that you've lost faith in them? Worrying that you'll upset them could be doing harm to yourself."

Tears filled my eyes.

"I think this may be what's causing your panic attacks, Sandi. I'll teach you how to stop them, but you're going to have to walk through the fire and feel the pain, no matter how frightening it gets. It's not going to be easy."

"You really think I'm having panic attacks? This would mean that after all these years, even after being told I'm going to die five times, that my body has finally reached the maximum amount of stress that it can handle. Plus, I do feel my feelings. I get angry."

"Actually, anger is a way people deflect what they're feeling."

Having a brain tumor and living for years with what felt like a ticking time bomb in my head—and now for a second time—had not been easy. Getting radiation damage on top of this had been particularly tough. Having three baffled neurologists who couldn't help me, at the same time my family had been spewing unrelenting anger ... I was being pushed over the edge.

A week after this appointment, I asked my doctors, "Is there anything I can do to help myself? If oxygen needs to get up into my brain, I'll stand on my head all day if you think it will help."

"There's nothing you can do," one doctor said.

I interpreted this as meaning that I had to find a way on my own. As my mother's anxiety worsened, the more she pressured my siblings. The more overwhelmed they both became, the more they all demanded the impossible from me.

After my brother yelled, "Get her off our backs," I finally understood that my siblings had been expecting and demanding I somehow make our emotionally unstable mother stable. And their stress had to be affecting their ability to think.

Rather than empathize with my grave situation, my family's anger continued to spiral. The solution to their problems, as my life fell apart, was to repeatedly demand that I end their suffering for them.

What contributed to my problems, which I will admit I created when I was a child, was that I'd always viewed my family in a flattering light. I decided if I could get them to calmly talk, our relationships would improve. I was sure that soon they would realize how callous and illogical they were acting, but the more I tried to talk to them, the more their anger escalated.

No matter how often I asked them what I did that made them so angry, none of them would tell me. At first, I thought I must have done something. There was even a time when I thought perhaps the brain tumor had caused me not to remember something that I did to them.

Because I loved my family, I fought hard to understand how they acted, until a time came when I no longer could deny that my family had serious emotional deficiencies. After a while I was able to see that their problems started long before I got sick. Intellectually, I understood this, but letting go of the people I had always believed them to be proved to be far more difficult.

***

64

"You won't believe what she did this time," I overheard my mother telling my sister on the phone.

As much as I hate to eavesdrop, I'm finally going to find out what the problem is.

"And in my own home. I can't take this any longer. I gave her a roof over her head and food to eat and all she does is scream at me," she said, before bursting into tears.

What my mother said made no sense. I hadn't yelled at her. Lying was something she had always done. (We used to call it exaggerating or fibbing, to be kind.) And yet both my siblings believed her? And why, only after I got radiation damage, did my family turn on me? Why not seven years before when I was diagnosed with the brain tumor? Why did they wait?

Because before, I didn't need their help, and now I did. It was only after my mother insisted on coming to the hospital, and told me not to take Gainor, that her emotional state deteriorated and these problems began. Clearly, my mother was orchestrating this. Pitting her three children against one another was nothing new.

I remembered the time decades before when I was sitting naked in the bathtub, young enough to still be bathed. My mother leaned over and whispered, "You are so beautiful, but don't tell your sister because she'll get angry at you."

I thought, *but how can I hide my face? How can I be comfortable in front of my sister ever again?*

My mother had to have seen the look of panic on my young, innocent face. She must have seen how uncomfortable I had become. What the child in me didn't realize was that my mother was creating a bond between us while creating a division between my sister and me. She had convinced me that she was my protector, and manipulated me so she and only she would be the receiver of my love.

My mother was so desperate to be loved that she wanted her children to love her, but not one another. My two siblings, who were older than me, saw through her tactics when they were young. Shortly after graduating from college, my sister told me, "I considered getting married in high school just to get out of the house because I resented that the adults in our home weren't acting like adults."

After my brother graduated from college, he moved to Africa, where he lived for a long time, getting as far away from our mother as he could. During the time of Beatlemania when almost every young man grew his hair long, she had nagged him for growing his, and used to call him a "homo." So why were both my siblings believing her now and not me?

***

Years before I got sick, I heard my sister refer to our biological father as emotionally retarded. And yet she never noticed that she struggled emotionally, too? And my mother and siblings thought it was healthy to hold on to their anger year after year?

While still living with my mother, I began getting what I thought were excruciating full-body migraines that left me exhausted for days. When one occurred, like a heavy New England snowstorm, everything came to a halt.

People React to Our Getting Sick Based on Their Experience

Take nothing anyone says or does personally—ever. If you haven't read or even if you have, read the book The Four Agreements *by don Miguel Ruiz, specifically the chapter titled, "Don't Take Anything Personally." Here, the author explains that when you take anything personally, this poisons you. Nothing anyone does is because of you.*

Whenever you get upset about anything, notice if this is because you've taken something personally.

Write down every time you notice you have taken something personally and what this cost you.

_____

_____

_____

_____

_____

_____

_____

_____

Write down the times you refused to take something personally.

_____

_____

_____

_____

_____

_____

_____

_____

11

The Effects of Being Appreciative
Will Surprise You

Viktor Frankl, an Austrian neurologist, psychiatrist, philosopher, Holocaust survivor, and author of one of my favorite books, *Man's Search for Meaning*, studied prisoners in Auschwitz. He determined that our thoughts affect our lives, and when our appreciation is greater than our fears, our lives become significantly affected in positive ways.

I empowered myself by taking responsibility for my thoughts, actions, and feelings. Whenever I got emotionally triggered, I used this to my benefit by asking, "How else might I look at this? What can I learn from the way I reacted?" Keeping the focus strictly on myself, and not on another's offensive behavior, gave me useful information that I used to understand and strengthen myself.

Years before, to keep from being manipulated by Gary, every time he tried to start a fight, I learned to not react by taking a breath and grounding myself. I'd hoped that using this same technique with my mother and siblings would stop the migraines, but nothing I did helped.

In the organization, Adult Children of Alcoholics (ACOA), we are called adult children because we grew up in homes where there was substance abuse. Because we had no healthy role models when we were young, we have a challenging time maturing emotionally. My siblings and I were no exceptions.

Having never gone to 12-step meetings or gotten counseling to help themselves, my siblings reacted to my getting sick and needing my family's support in the only way they knew. As children, they saw our mother get angry and blame others, so they responded in this same way. To them, this was normal.

68

Our mother didn't know how to regulate her nervous system, which contributed to her emotional instability and "drama queen" behavior. My siblings held onto their anger year after year because this is what our mother did.

It took me years of pain and confusion, while I also struggled with my health, before I could understand that it was from the pain my mother and my siblings felt—due to their inability to regulate their nervous systems—that caused them to turn on me. Once I understood the severity of their emotional challenges and the pain and devastation that they experienced, I couldn't help but feel sorry for them. My hurt and confusion turned to compassion, which also contributed to the strengthening of my body.

Because they falsely believed I had caused their problems, the idea of coming to my aid and supporting me was impossible. Due to their overwhelming emotions, they couldn't think rationally and consider the tremendous amount of stress on me, and that it was barbaric to be contributing to this.

Our father dealt with his problems by drinking. Our mother reacted to her problems by becoming overly dramatic, manipulating others to get their help, and medicating herself when things got tough. It is no surprise my siblings and I grew up with poor emotional coping skills. And because the three of us witnessed our parents struggling with trust issues, trust was challenging for us as well.

After I was diagnosed with radiation damage, my family's emotional restrictions festered. None of them knew to ask, "What can I learn about myself by how I'm reacting?" or "How might I benefit by seeing things differently?" Instead, they acted as they had been taught to act: They got angry and blamed me for their pain and helplessness.

They lacked the ability to look at themselves. They accepted how angry and cruel they behaved. They failed to see that I was just the catalyst that exposed the emotional challenges they already had. They missed the opportunity to learn from this to become emotionally mature and create a far less challenging life for themselves. And today, I still grieve this.

My role, as the baby in the family, had long been established by the time I got sick. As is often expected of the youngest, I was to behave, learn from, and mimic my elders, just as I had always done growing up. But I no longer could. When five neurologists couldn't save my life, I had to change so I could live. Unwelcomed changes within any family will create stress. My family's anger and resentment flared like a hot lit match.

Empowering Yourself

I empowered myself by taking responsibility for my thoughts, actions, and feelings. I expanded my thinking and knowledge by asking how else I might look at each of my challenges. By keeping the focus on myself, and not on another's offensive behavior and blaming others for my behavior whenever I got triggered, I used what this revealed about myself to gain strength. Lori had taught me that our immune systems work most efficiently when we're happy. Because I wanted to heal myself, I knew being happy would help me.

Make a list of ways you empower yourself and write the ways you can teach yourself to become more empowered.

_____

_____

_____

_____

_____

_____

_____

What ways do you give yourself and your power away? What does this cost you? What ways might you change to empower yourself?

_____

_____

_____

_____

_____

_____

_____

_____

12

Coping with Others' Reactions

"In the African tradition, mothers are to be respected no matter what!" my brother yelled, expecting me to follow a tradition from another culture just because he used to live there and he chose to follow this. How can someone so worldly think in such a restricted way? My sister accused me of "breaking up the family" and yet it was she, my brother, and our mother who turned on me. Even though I kept telling everyone in my family that I only wanted peace, none of them could see through their illogical thinking. I found this to be quite scary.

According to my mother, both of my siblings had chosen the "wrong person" to marry years before. My brother wasn't supposed to marry a Black woman from Africa, and my sister was supposed to marry someone who was more educated. My mother cried for months about this and leaned on me for support, which naturally I had given her. So, both of my siblings knew what it was like to be on the receiving end of our mother's wrath. Only they knew the extent of our mother's relentlessness and why I was desperate for their help.

For the past year, my mother had been demanding that the two of us discuss the selling of her house. I had no idea why she was insisting I be included in this conversation. For reasons I didn't yet understand, every time she brought this subject up, I had a full-blown panic attack. Feeling like my life was threatened, I ran from the room to save my life.

"You know Mom likes it when others make decisions for her, so she doesn't have to take responsibility. And you know she gets brutal if she doesn't get her way," my sister said after I told her I felt like I would die whenever Mom brought this subject up. So my sister knew that Mom could be brutal, and she knew that I was struggling with my health and having panic attacks. And yet she still wouldn't help me. Why?

Our mother had convinced my siblings that I was the reason for her emotional decline; that she desperately needed their help to protect her from me. Through tears and guilt, she managed to manipulate them into being loyal to her, just as she had done to me when I was young and didn't know better.

To hold on to her control, my mother kept pouring gas into this emotional inferno. I saw her doing this, but there was nothing I could do to stop her from lying about me and exploiting the love of her two oldest children. And I couldn't stop my siblings from believing her, no matter how hard I tried. Everyone's anger and frustrations were amplified as my mother delighted in creating this drama.

On Thanksgiving Day in 1998, my mother and I were seated at the Seaman's Inn restaurant on the grounds of the Mystic Seaport Museum, just miles from our home. I was enjoying the holiday smells that permeated around me in this lovely historical setting. I loved smelling the combination of turkey, sage stuffing, and cranberry sauce, with just a hint of apple pie that lingered in the air.

I was thrilled to have this rare opportunity to relax and enjoy my mother's company, just like I used to do not that many years ago. I looked across the table at her classic beauty and her gorgeous green eyes that changed color depending on what she wore. Ever since I was a little girl, this had delighted and fascinated me. The green silk dress she wore looked stunning on her, but her jaw was tightly clenched.

To help her relax, I smiled. She turned her head and scanned the room. I attempted to make small talk, but she showed no interest. As soon as we ordered our meals, she leaned across the table and said, "Now you have no choice. You have to talk to me about selling the house."

My stomach turned and my body trembled from this unexpected sneak attack. "Mom, please don't do this. It's Thanksgiving. Let's talk about things we're grateful for. I, for one, am grateful I have this opportunity to enjoy Thanksgiving with you. Who knows how many more Thanksgivings we'll get to spend together?"

"Grateful?! You've got to be kidding. Do you know how many times you've refused to have this conversation?"

"Yes, I do, and every time I told you I can't discuss this. You must be able to hear the nervousness in my voice, see the fear on my face, and how anxious I get every time you bring this up. I wish I could talk to you about this. I really do, but as I've explained to you many times, I always get a panic attack for reasons I can't explain."

"So, you're still using that same old excuse?"

I paused, realizing that she was leaving me with no choice. "Unless you're willing to enjoy this holiday with me, as I trusted when you invited me to have dinner with you, I'm going to leave. I don't want to have a panic attack in public, Mom."

Her clamped jaw and the glaring anger in her eyes revealed that she was not giving up. My heart was beating rapidly as I slid my wooden thumb-back chair away from the table. I took a deep breath and waited a moment while never taking my eyes off of my mother. I stood and held the chair's top rail to keep myself from falling while I waited for my mother to tell me to sit back down.

She raised her chin as if to say, "You wouldn't dare." I waited a moment longer before I turned and walked towards the front door, hoping to hear her call my name.

Outside, it was dark and raining. The cool winter air felt good against my warm reddened face. I had driven us to the restaurant, so I had the car keys. Because I had gotten wet crossing the large parking lot, I welcomed the protection the car now offered. To avoid getting a migraine, I leaned against the steering wheel and tried to relax.

To be in the presence of anyone who showed no regard for my welfare was unhealthy. I had no choice but to leave. A part of me wanted to drive away and leave my mother here, but I refused to let her ruthlessness change who I was. I wouldn't be as cruel as she was. Over 11 years earler, in January 1987, I chose to use love as my guide and had done my best to be as faithful as I could to this. I wasn't about to stop now.

"Love doesn't mean being a doormat, Sandi. You need to act as loving towards yourself as you are towards others," Lori had repeatedly told me, but because this was not how I'd been raised, this was a hard habit to break. Obviously, my mother expected me to be her doormat, but this was too unhealthy. I needed to help my body heal.

But I did it! Having a panic attack in a public place no doubt would have meant I was allowing myself to be walked on again. I had set a boundary like Lori had taught me. And I certainly had given my mother fair warning in a kind and respectful way.

No one can afford to be emotionally abused, yet my mother seemed to think she had a right to mistreat me. Lori had to keep reminding me that for my body to heal, I had to protect myself from my mother's melodrama, especially since the migraines had gotten worse.

She was still my mother, and she deserved for me to wait and drive her home, regardless of how cruelly she treated me. After all, she gave me life. Maybe by now, she realized that sabotaging her daughter on Thanksgiving Day is not how mothers were supposed to act.

Minutes later, the passenger door opened. My mother climbed in soaking wet. Her hair was stuck to her head, causing it to look odd and misshapen. Dark mascara was smeared over her glaring eyes. An ugly black line streamed down one cheek. I'd never seen my mother look this repugnant before.

Bitterly, she glared and said, "I hope you feel good about yourself for ruining my Thanksgiving."

Stop Trying to Change or Control Others

Trying to control others is unhealthy, and creates stress and unhappiness. My brother wanted me to follow an African tradition because he did. Because my siblings married people my mother didn't approve of, she made herself miserable. My siblings wanted me to make our emotionally unstable mother stable, which only brought all of us misery.

Write down every time you accepted and respected another's right to live their life the way they chose even though you did not agree with their choice.

_____

_____

_____

_____

_____

_____

_____

_____

Write down each time you notice that you attempted to change someone and the result. What did this cost you?

_____

_____

_____

_____

_____

_____

_____

_____

13

Using Anger to Your Advantage

Driving two hours north on I-95 from Connecticut to Massachusetts General Hospital in Boston had gotten old and tiresome. I had been making this trip at least twice a month for almost two years and I was not getting better. My three neurosurgeons continued to discuss solutions to my problems because they didn't know what to do. Since I knew my body well, I yearned to share my perspective, but all three doctors discouraged me from talking at all. Sitting on the sidelines had never been a strength of mine.

How could my confidence in them not have faded? Since I had no health insurance, and they and the hospital had volunteered their services, my options were pretty limited. Adding to my frustrations, I had been told that the second medication, Trental, had no side effects, but my body had proved them wrong.

Since 1986, after being told I would soon die, I continued to be traumatized—when I got radiation damage; when I learned part of the AVM was still in my head and I could possibly die again any second; and by my family's anger and betrayal the very first time I needed their help.

The migraines had become more frequent, intense, and painful and were often happening multiple times each week. My mother seemed to enjoy igniting my panic attacks. She knew the migraines were influenced by stress, so why was she seemingly trying to cause one every chance she got?

Standing on the beach, just two blocks from my home, I closed my eyes and turned to feel the warm sun on my face and asked, *What am I to do now?* Clearly, I heard a voice inside tell me, *Try a different approach.*

I found what I needed from Dr. Deirdre O'Connor, a highly respected local naturopathic physician who practiced just 10 minutes from my home. She offered her services to me for free. When I told her I felt like I was dying on Trental, she read out loud from a large reference book. This medication had never been tested on menstruating women and cancer was a possible side effect.

"You have got to be kidding me! You won't believe the sexism I've experienced in the medical world. All I want is to get better. And now I could get cancer, too? No wonder my body's rejecting this medication."

Dr. O'Connor explained that I could get the same results my doctors were trying to achieve by taking fish oil supplements and eating copious amounts of salmon, mackerel, sardines, and herring. "Because your Dutch ancestors ate a diet that included lots of fish, I'm not surprised that your body is asking for this in order to heal itself."

"You really think this will work?"

"According to the *New England Journal of Medicine*, there's been excellent results. And fish oil has no side effects."

"I've gotten side effects from the medications used to treat the side effects I got from my original treatment. I really need to break this cycle and free myself from this ongoing craziness."

"This is the problem with our allopathic health care I've seen way too often. I think you've suffered long enough, don't you?"

"I'd be foolish if I didn't give my immune system a chance to do what it was created to do. Plus, I like the idea that because my ancestors ate a lot of fish, that fish oil can now help me. That's really cool."

When I got home, I looked to see if Trental had any other side effects and found these listed: drowsiness (check), headaches (check), insomnia (check), muscle aches (check), agitation and anxiety (check).

I had them all. I was so furious I decided I would walk into my next appointment in Boston naked, so my doctors had to notice I was a female. Once my anger subsided, I decided wearing a pink dress would get my point across.

When I next went to Boston, I handed one of the doctors the article from the *New England Journal of Medicine* that Dr. O'Connor had given me to give them, proving that fish oil successfully thins blood. Seconds later, one doctor leaped towards me, shook his finger in my face and shouted, "You had better not be thinking of going off this medication!"

I had thought we could still work together, but since I chose not to take the medication they prescribed I was no longer welcomed? I asked how long I was expected to remain on Trental.

"For the rest of your life," Dr. Shaky Finger said.

I had never been told this before. If doctors—or anyone—weren't willing to work *with* me, how could I possibly work with them? All relationships, by definition, require at least some attempt to be made at relating, and yet there are people, including brain surgeons, who don't understand or practice this.

I cried as I drove the two hours home, knowing I would never take Trental again. I grieved for all the time I had invested and for the faith I lost. Because I put my trust in these doctors, I had given up my home and moved in with my mother, which became the lowest and most miserable point in my life. I followed Dr. O'Connor's natural approach and, although the migraines continued, my body thrived under her care.

Because of my frustrating and costly experience, I suggest others first look for a natural substance that works as well as or even better than any prescribed medication.

Elyn Jacobs, a certified cancer coach, strategist, and a two-time breast cancer survivor wrote in her blog: "Prescription drugs are the third leading cause of death after heart disease and cancer, and most come with the risk of potentially toxic side effects and contribute to further disease, not wellness; drugs do not cure imbalances, they create them."

I walked away from three respected neurosurgeons who generously volunteered their time and expertise to help me, who were working at a hospital ranked among the top hospitals in America by *U.S. News & World Report*. My body told me I needed a different kind of care than what they offered, and thankfully, I listened. If I had known then what I know now, I could have avoided the most painful, challenging, and frightening years of my life.

Today, I am elated to report that Massachusetts General Hospital not only offers comprehensive and integrated health care, but is one of the leading hospitals in our nation that does. They have learned that it's important for their doctors to work with their patients; that every patient's body must be treated individually. They now know that not only do patients have the right to participate in their own health care, but when doctors and patients work together, patients get the best care.

I spent decades teaching myself to interpret the language my body speaks. I recommend that everyone learn to understand theirs beginning now, before their health fails. Like a mother who understands her baby's individual cries, everyone can become accustomed to their body's many voices and learn what their body is saying it needs. The more time I took to understand mine, the easier it became to interpret, and the more amazed I was at its intelligence. Know that your body is always coming from a place of love. Despite experiencing a high level of physical pain, I can still say that our bodies are never revengeful or cruel. They are always doing their best to help us. And since our immune systems work most efficiently when we're happy, fulfilling our hearts' desires helps our bodies to thrive. So follow your bliss and be led by love.

A doctor may be excellent, but my experience has proven that no one can afford to consider their doctor as a god. If you were to go to an art auction, you would see a wide variety of art for sale. You might love some of these paintings and others you wouldn't hang in your home if you were paid a million dollars. This is because we are all individuals, and our doctors need to treat us as such.

People like and dislike different kinds of foods. We buy various types and colors of cars. Some of us sleep with the window open, while others do not like this at all. We think nothing of how our bodies respond when we listen to music we love or when we decorate our homes. Our bodies tell us when we're hungry and thirsty, when we've gotten too much sun, when to turn our thermostat up or down, and when we want sex or don't.

So why is it a stretch to listen to our bodies when it comes to our medical care?

Trusting Your Body's Wisdom

When my body told me to try a different approach, I knew to listen. It was no coincidence that my body responded to a natural remedy that provided my brain with the oxygen it needed. I had been driving a two-hour round trip to Boston to be treated using medicines that my body fought. When the three doctors were unwilling to work with me and I was expected to be on their medication forever, it became clear my body had been protecting me from harm and wanted me to go in a different direction.

Write down each time you did what your body told you to do and the outcome. (Eating, sleeping, having sex, etc. may be left off this list.)

_____

_____

_____

_____

_____

_____

And keep a list of every time you decided not to listen to what your body told you and the results from this. What did this cost you?

_____

_____

_____

_____

_____

_____

_____

14

Taking a Vacation Can Give You Perspective

While I was inching my way towards better health, my mother's emotional state continued to unravel. My siblings became more frantic and each of them put more pressure on me. To escape this ongoing madness, I applied and received a month-long scholarship to a holistic teachers' program at the Kripalu Center for Yoga and Health in the beautiful Berkshire Mountains, just a three-hour drive north of my home.

Though I had been following Lori and Dr. O'Connor's advice, the migraines had continued to worsen in both pain and frequency. I suspected the stress was from my mother's ongoing deterioration and her daily aggressions were agitating them.

I was scared to go away in my weakened state, but I was more afraid if the migraines continued to get worse. If I didn't get a break from the toxic environment I was living in, I feared I would be stuck living with my mother for the rest of my life.

Was my mother using me, purposely keeping me sick, needing me to live with her to give purpose to her life?

Like a heavy rain after a lengthy drought, Kripalu brought me the peaceful, supportive atmosphere my body yearned for. It was exactly what I needed. From the safety it gave me, I could feel my body relax as my nervous system calmed and regulated itself, allowing me to think more clearly.

It was here that I did one of the hardest things I've ever done. I reviewed a conversation I'd had with my mother as I was leaving home. It was this that made me realize if she and my siblings chose not to share their love with me, I had to accept this. It was gut-wrenching and painful to face the fact that I no longer had a family whose love I could always count on.

Since they chose to act like my enemies, I had to let them be, as hard as this was. For the sake of my health, I had no choice. The most loving thing I could do for us all was to stop resisting the choices they made and allow them to live however they chose, which is what I had wanted from them.

"I understand it must be terribly frightening for a mother to see her child struggling with her health. I'm sorry you've had to go through this," I said to my mother just as I was about to drive to Kripalu.

"It sure has been hell for me. But what are you really saying, Sandi? You can't be trusted, so there's got to be more to this."

No one had ever accused me of being untrustworthy before. "I'm just saying that I can see you're in a lot of pain and I'm sorry. We both thought my health problems were long behind me, but in many ways, they keep getting worse. I know this has been hard on both of us."

"You have no idea of how difficult this is for me, so don't stand there acting like you know just to make yourself feel better before you go off and enjoy yourself."

"I understand that no one can know exactly what another is feeling. I'm just saying I'm sorry that you're in pain, too."

"Too? Now I get it. You're trying to manipulate me to get my attention on you, while you're appearing to be so sweet and innocent. I'm onto the tricks you're always playing."

It is clear who the game player is, I thought as I climbed into my car. But why? What happened to create this distorted version of my once loving mother?

***

Practicing yoga six mornings each week for the entire month I was at Kripalu felt luxurious. It made my body feel alive again and trained me to focus inwardly to find the solace my body craved. Being at Kripalu and hiking in the Berkshires nurtured my body, mind, and spirit by saturating me with tender love and support. By the end of the month, I felt my emotional equilibrium had vastly improved, which helped me to acquire more patience and resilience—skills I would need for the challenges ahead.

Despite attempting to create a similar peaceful and supportive environment once I returned home, my mother told me I had no right to try to change anything in the house she owned. To regain some independence, I got a job in a bakery on the grounds of the Mystic Seaport Museum.

Just as I was about to walk out the door to drive to work during my second week, my mother, still dressed in her pink velour bathrobe, her brown hair disheveled, yelled, "I loved my life while you were away! I had peace with you gone!"

Faced with the reality that my mother truly hated me, something in me shattered. I cried on my way to work. After being on my feet for hours, a migraine erupted, forcing me to leave while I could still drive home. Since I couldn't promise my boss that this wouldn't happen again, I got fired from a job for the first time in my life. I was embarrassed, humiliated, ashamed, and discouraged by yet another loss the brain tumor had caused. I feared I was never going to get a foundation, the momentum I needed to reestablish my life.

And the fact that I lost my job infuriated my mother. I didn't take this setback well either. I couldn't even hold a job selling oatmeal and chocolate chip cookies? My mother took advantage of my vulnerable state just like Gary used to do, insisting that we discuss selling her house. The panic attacks flourished, and the migraines increased. I spent most of the next two weeks recuperating by taking hot baths or lying in bed.

"Did you notice that you never had a migraine or a panic attack while you were at Kripalu? You now have proof that how your mother treats you affects your body," Lori pointed out at my next appointment.

"But I can't live at Kripalu, as much as I wish I could."

"Do you think it would be helpful if you set more boundaries?"

Like a determined two-year-old, my mother fought back against every boundary I set.

I had learned a lot about addictions from living with Gary and attending 12-step meetings. So when I saw a job advertised in the newspaper regarding addiction prevention, I got an interview and got the job.

I was to teach drug and alcohol prevention workshops at the Naval Submarine Base in Groton, about 25 minutes from my home, to young, bright submariners who were enthusiastic and welcoming. As my experience grew (and my body adapted), my schedule would increase. It was a perfect fit for me.

I received two weeks of training, which I loved. I studied hard. I enjoyed being part of a team that worked well together. I had 25 students in my first workshop and received 100 percent positive feedback from all of them and my boss. My spirit was ignited until, just before I was scheduled to teach my second workshop, another migraine forced me to bed.

I let a lot of people down and inconvenienced many. Because I couldn't promise that I could be relied on to work when needed, I lost this job, too.

My mother screamed in anger when I told her. Before my body got completely drained and I went insane, I made an appointment with a doctor to get a prescription to stop the migraines. Regardless of how my body responded, I had to stop them from ruining my life.

"Your migraines aren't exactly what I'd call migraines," this primary care physician said. "The radiation damage is what's causing the pain. Your nervous system relays messages to and from your brain through your spinal cord down to your toes, which is why you have pain all throughout your body, and why you're left exhausted for days."

Well, at least someone understands.

"It's not uncommon after having a migraine for someone's body to feel pummeled, but because of the radiation damage, you keep getting extra wallops. The damage to your pons makes fixing this problem even more complex."

Once again, this persnickety pons is causing problems.

"I seriously doubt what you have are migraines, but if you're comfortable calling them this ... Just know it's my responsibility to tell you that I think what you have goes way beyond just a migraine."

No wonder the pain has been so intense.

"And you're also resistant to medications because of your body's sensitivity to drugs, most likely due to the damage to your pons."

Interesting ...

"But these so-called migraines have been keeping you from having a life. It may take a while before we find the right medication. I do have to warn you that things may get worse before they get better."

Worse? I've been losing years of my life because of these migraines or whatever the hell I'm supposed to call them—radiation damage reactors? While my friends have been establishing their careers, settling down and getting married, traveling, or having kids, I've been lying in my bathtub or bed for hours.

***

"So, the first medication didn't work. We'll try another," this doctor replied when I saw him next.

"No. I can't go through that again! I thought I was dying. I even asked my mother to come and sit with me because I didn't want to die alone, but she left the room after less than a minute because she couldn't cope with what was happening to me."

***

Having the best of mother nature at my doorstep and going on long, relaxing walks brought me precious pockets of relief. I loved hearing the sounds of the seagulls calling out as if to make me smile and cheer me on. The salt air and the wide-open expanse of water made me feel safe and cared for, tucked into nature's loving arms. Walking along the shoreline gave me the nurturing I craved for and couldn't get at home.

Often, I would sit on East Dock where I used to fish when I was young and just watch the waves as they broke all along the shore, mesmerized by their rhythmic consistency and their gentle soothing sounds.

When I left home each day, I never knew if I would find the water calm and smooth, reflecting the white sails of the sailboats, or if she would be flexing her muscles and chopping at the water, and only old, weathered workboats would dare be out.

Some days, the water appeared to demand my attention: she would lift herself up high above the water's surface, splashing about in all directions before falling back down with a loud fluid crash.

I was thrilled whenever the wind caught small droplets of salt water and tossed them in the air. As if she knew my energy was lacking and my spirit battered, Mother Nature would kiss my cheek with a cool and loving water droplet. I grinned with delight, like a little kid.

When I religiously practiced the stress management tools Lori taught me, didn't push myself too hard, and I avoided my mother's aggression as best I could, my body grew stronger step by step. Often, I got exactly what I needed from a casual conversation.

"Are you familiar with the Zen way of thinking?" Gainor asked me in the studio we shared while pushing her short, snow-white hair from her face. "Trying too hard and doing too much can work against us. You're working hard so you can move out of your mother's house, but you're putting even more stress on yourself."

"I have to move as soon as possible. She's driving me crazy."

"If you had a boss who worked you as hard as you do, you would have quit long ago. Because I see you almost every day, I feel it's my responsibility to say something. When was the last time you took a day off since you got back from Kripalu?"

And from Lori, I heard, "Because your family expects you to get better faster than your body can heal, I see you keep pushing yourself. You have accepted a lot about your family already, but your concern for them and what they think may still be doing your body harm. By pushing yourself, do you think you may be making it more difficult to hear your body's wisdom?"

I had hoped, when I first moved in with my mother, that I would have been able to help her as well, since her husband had died the year before and she hadn't been the same since. I thought her grief was causing her decline, but now I knew there had to be more to it.

When we lived together from the fall of 1994 to June 1999, I had no idea why my mother had changed so drastically and why her love for me turned to hatred. Or why she became so aggressive and tried to make me miserable every day.

The Healing Power of Nature

When you are outside walking, notice what you are seeing, hearing, and smelling. Notice how your breathing slows down and how much calmer you feel. Walking can help protect us from heart disease, depression, anxiety, attention disorder, and many other imbalances. Nature gives us a break from the hectic world we live in because nature is not demanding of us.

Next time you're feeling stressed, anxious, or depressed, go for a walk. Or, better yet, go before to decrease your chances of becoming stressed.

Write down how you felt before and after your walk. And notice how you feel when you haven't been outdoors for a long while.

_____

_____

_____

_____

_____

_____

_____

_____

_____

_____

_____

_____

_____

_____

_____

_____

15

The Effects from Being Traumatized

If my mother kept demanding we discuss the selling of her house and the migraines kept getting worse, why had I not acquiesced to having this talk?

My mother had insisted she come with me when I returned to Massachusetts General Hospital to get my test results. Both of us heard my doctor say I had radiation damage, and a part of the AVM was still in my head and could be life-threatening.

What made this frightening prognosis even more agonizing was hearing my mother screaming about my possible death while I was still trying to assimilate my doctor's words. Hearing that I was in possible danger of dying in seconds again left me raw and vulnerable. My mother yelling about my possible dying forced me to face this before I was emotionally able. Yelling about selling her house and my death became enmeshed inside me, where this trauma remained buried.

Until my mother insisted we discuss her house being sold, this had remained dormant and undisturbed. But her constant persistence brought what felt like life-threatening terror to the surface. Every time she demanded that we have this talk, she uprooted this. She watched me panic and run in fear for my life as she repeatedly tortured me. She appeared to enjoy having this control over me and seeing me panic. Loving the feeling of power this gave her, she didn't stop this torture for years.

I begged her to stop. I told my two siblings I was in desperate need of their help, but my mother continued to toy with my fear of death. Between her aggression and my siblings' anger I bottomed out emotionally and physically. If I had health insurance, I would have checked myself into the nearest psychiatric ward and been grateful to have the protection it offered.

In the decades ahead, I showed multiple signs of trauma: exhaustion, confusion, sadness, free-form anxiety, agitation, mistrust, and being on guard. I had trouble sleeping and concentrating. I lived with overwhelming shame and guilt. If things got too tough I "checked out" (what my therapist called "dissociating").

"Trauma comes back as a reaction, not a memory," wrote Bessel van der Kolk, one of the world's leading experts in the treatment of trauma and author of *The Body Keeps Score*. Because of my uncontrollable and often embarrassing reactions, I secluded myself in my home for years. I only went out in public when I felt safe.

Following the murder of George Floyd in 2020 by Derek Chauvin, a policeman who was supposed to be trustworthy and help people, I became highly agitated and didn't know why. It was a while before I understood, and it was only because I remembered a similar incident that happened six years before after the murder of Nicole Brown by (I believe) her ex-husband, someone she once loved and trusted.

My body reacted on a cellular level both times, long before I intellectually understood why I had become so anxious and fearful: I trusted and loved my mother and both my siblings, and yet all three of them had repeatedly traumatized me.

Setting Boundaries to Help You Heal

Learning to say no and setting boundaries are the limits you set regarding your time, emotions, body, and mental health. They help you stay resilient and grounded, and protect you from being used, drained, or manipulated by others. They also create clear communication by defining what you will and will not tolerate. Setting boundaries will help you take charge of your life, which is essential, especially after you are traumatized. Even if people don't respect a boundary you set, discovering who does and who doesn't is something I found helpful because it allowed me to see who was and who wasn't respecting me and my right to heal myself.

Keep a list of when you said no and whenever you set a boundary for yourself and how setting each boundary helped you.

_____

_____

_____

_____

Keep a list of who is not respecting your boundaries and how you might successfully navigate around this.

_____

_____

_____

_____

What ways did you fail and how might you improve in the future?

_____

_____

_____

_____

16

Your Responsibility is to Protect Yourself from Harm

A local reporter called, wanting to interview me after he heard I had radiation damage. Memories of what I once accomplished, what most artists only dream about, came flooding back to me. Katharine Hepburn's literary agent had courted me. I met her in New York and agreed to have her represent me, but when she learned I had radiation damage, she dropped me like a hot potato.

I enjoyed my conversation with this pleasant reporter, who treated me kindly and with respect. He asked provocative questions that were fun to answer. Without giving it any thought, I told him that part of the AVM had never left my head and could still be life-threatening, the first time I told this to anyone.

While I was reaching for a glass from the kitchen cupboard later that week, my mother stormed into the house screaming. Clenching the rolled-up newspaper in her hand, she stomped into the kitchen and pounded it on the counter just inches from where I stood.

"You're such a liar! What the hell is wrong with you? You told this reporter the AVM's still in your head? Are you that desperate for attention?"

Seeing my mother in such a frenzied state and hearing this bizarre accusation stunned me. I'd heard her scream when the doctor told us this. Never had I seen my mother, or anyone before, be this unruly and lose their dignity like this, unless they were intoxicated. I told her she would feel better once she relaxed, but this upset her even more.

Had the pressure of my illness pushed her too far and distorted her thinking to this extreme? Guilt tore through my body. I stepped back to assess her. The look of hatred in her eyes made my skin crawl. I was afraid I might be in danger. Leaning my right hip against the kitchen drawer where the knives were kept, I glanced around the room to assess the quickest exit.

From the look of loathing in her eyes, I understood why some people believe the devil can possess us. Particularly sickening was that her anger appeared to be exciting her. Once again, I tried to calm her, but I got the same rebellious, angry response as before. I decided it might be better for both of us if I just walked away.

While listening for sounds of her sneaking up behind me, I ascended the nearby stairs, hoping I wouldn't get stabbed in the back. Once safely inside my bedroom, I locked the door and collapsed on my bed.

My mother had convinced herself she had never heard the doctor say a part of the AVM was seen in my head. She thought I had to be a liar for telling the reporter this.

How could she believe that after 40 years I have suddenly started lying? And how could my siblings believe her, and not me, when she was known for lying?

I realized that how she was acting went way beyond anything I could have done. By reminding me of my possible death in such a diabolical manner, she obviously didn't care about killing me by making the AVM bleed. But why?

Had she and my siblings decided it would be easier on them if I were dead? Is this why they have all decided to gang up on me during the most vulnerable time in my life and taken turns attacking me for years? Wait a minute, who's acting crazy now?

None of them was thinking about me at all because they weren't capable of thinking beyond themselves.

What does this say about them?

I had such a difficult time accepting how emotionally challenged my family was. To see them in this different light was heart-wrenching, but seeing my mother in this frenzy opened up my eyes. It became clear I had to protect myself from all of them.

It's painful to think about the amount of pain they must be in, and how lost and misguided they had to be. Regardless of how they treated me, I didn't want this to be true. But why wouldn't they realize how unhealthy their behavior was and why didn't they get help for themselves? I didn't know which pain was greater—my own or realizing my family's mental state.

None of them could tell they weren't acting out of love?

I decided that my mother had to be the most wounded of the three, but since she had been able to get my siblings to follow her lead, what did that say about them? Since they couldn't see that they were enabling her, and making this problem worse for us all, what did it say about their lack of awareness?

After years of counseling, I now understood that my mother lacked the emotional ability to accept my diagnosis. When she was at the hospital her brain must have shut down to protect her, which blocked her from remembering what the doctor said. In her mind, I had to be an attention-grabbing liar.

I shudder to think that the same overwhelming terror my mother felt in the hospital when she'd screamed in fear of my death got triggered when she read the newspaper article—just as my terror was triggered every time she insisted we discuss the selling of her house.

Because she had insisted on coming to the hospital in Gainor's place, my mother never forgave me. And my siblings have never forgiven me for what they both believe I did to her.

At times, I still remind myself that if my mother had not loved me as much as she did, she never would have gotten as upset at the hospital. If she had allowed Gainor to come to support me, instead of insisting I take *her*, or if she had ever learned how to effectively cope with her emotions, her life, my life, and the lives of my siblings would never have been so emotionally turbulent.

If my mother had been capable of doing the appropriate thing, comforting me, her daughter, after I learned I had radiation damage and could again die in seconds, our relationship would never have deteriorated like it did. If I had thought about my needs and not put my mother's desires before my own, I can only imagine how much quicker my healing would have been.

My mother couldn't consider me any more than Gary could after I told him I had a brain tumor because they were both hijacked by their feelings. Even though my mother had never accused me of lying before, her emotions distorted her thinking and made her believe whatever she had to believe in order to protect herself. Seeing how she responded to the newspaper article, I now understood why she had to convince herself I was a horrible person who deserved to be punished for the pain I caused. And to my horror, punish me she did. And she persuaded my siblings to believe what she falsely believed. Out of loyalty to her, they both responded with vengeance, while my mother planned her own revenge. I only wanted peace, to be left alone to heal, but every time I expressed this, my mother pursued me more.

It got so bad I had to put a stop to this. I couldn't ignore it any longer.

"You can believe whatever you want about me, Mom. I know I'm innocent and my heart is pure."

She jumped back in a theatrical manner, staring wide-eyed at me, as if she'd seen a ghost. Acting like she was on stage before a large admiring audience, she yelled, "The machine did this to you! The cyclotron did this! You're not the daughter I once loved."

I froze. Tears streamed down my face, the only thing that moved in the room. Did she really say she no longer loved me, and the treatment had damaged my brain?

My mother laughed with glistening excitement as she studied my dazed expression.

"That's the cruelest thing anyone has ever said to me, Mom," I whispered, barely able to speak.

Driving aimlessly in my car, I wondered if there could be any truth to what she said. The problem with gaslighting, as she had been doing to me, was that it distorted my sense of reality. My ability to trust myself was nearly eroded.

If there really is something wrong with me, why did she yell this? Why is she so determined to break me while all my friends have been cheering me on and pointing to my progress with admiration?

When I returned home, my mother said in a calm and caring manner that I needed help, even if I didn't realize it yet.

"You've chosen to live in anger for years, and you've convinced both my siblings to follow your lead. And you think this is healthy?" I asked.

"Don't you dare speak to me like that in my own home!"

"You've used your children as pawns to get what you want, but I refuse to be bitter and angry like the three of you. God didn't create us to live in anger year after year after year."

To her credit, my mother began seeing a counselor. Just weeks later, she announced that I was to see this woman for just one visit because there were things my mother wanted me to know.

The counselor told me that my mother referred to me as "her happy and sensitive child who had a big heart, who always used to look after her." She wanted me to know that because no one ever treated my mother as lovingly as I had, my mother now had expectations of me that were impossible to fulfill. She warned me that my mother's anger had been building all her life because of the number of losses she had that she couldn't accept. What the counselor thought was particularly important for me to know was that all of my mother's lifelong anger was now being directed at me and I needed to protect myself.

I called my sister as soon as I got home to tell her Mom's anger wasn't my fault, but she showed no interest. Later, I offered to talk with my mother about what the counselor said.

"I paid her to talk to you because, obviously, I don't want to discuss it. Try to get that through that damaged brain of yours."

Knowing Who You Can't Afford to Be With

People can get hijacked by their feelings and imprisoned by them. But you are responsible for yourself: You must determine who is being rational and who has lost this ability. In this chapter, I explained how shocked and emotionally divided I was because I loved my mother. Fortunately, I had learned I had to be responsible for myself. Had I not protected myself, I hate to imagine what might have happened to me. Do not engage with people who do not care about hurting you or others.

Make a list of people in your life who get hijacked by their emotions, so you have this information to help you avoid being shocked when they become irrational, and you can protect yourself from them. Write down the times you purposely didn't engage when someone was being irrational.

_____

_____

_____

_____

_____

_____

Write down the times you tried talking with someone who was imprisoned by their feelings. How did this work out for you? And what did this cost you?

_____

_____

_____

_____

_____

_____

_____

17

People Don't Change Just Because You Get Sick

I don't remember exactly when I decided our Creator must have given us free will for a reason. I only know that out of respect for this, never again would I tell another adult what to do. But I was the only one in my family who thought like this.

About a month after seeing my mother's counselor, she announced, "I'm tired of playing this game of yours. You are to see my lawyer this afternoon." Though I had no idea why I was being told to go, I went, hoping I would learn something useful. After I introduced myself to this attorney, I sat in a chair opposite her large wooden desk. I expected our appointment to begin with her introducing herself and graciously thanking me for coming, but she only sat and glared at me.

Little did this woman know that I had been teaching myself not to be intimidated by others by studying how anger distorts a face. I decided this was a perfect time to practice this. As if I was about to paint her portrait, I sat and studied her strained facial muscles, and they began to twitch. The more I analyzed her, the more her muscles spasmed. To have some extra fun, I leaned across her wide desk to give myself a closer look. I continued studying her as if she had the most fascinating face I had ever seen. Amused by myself, I couldn't help but giggle.

"What's so funny?" this woman snapped.

"The way you've chosen to introduce yourself."

"Your mother says you're not working because you have migraines. I get migraines too and I work. So, what's your problem?"

This woman thinks I'll discuss my medical problems with her? And she thinks our migraines are comparable?

I had come here with good intentions, hoping to get some insight that might improve my relationship with my mother, not to engage in this lawyer's eccentricities.

Lori had taught me that no one had a right to treat me disrespectfully under any circumstances. By this time, I had been doing everything I could to assist my body's healing for almost ten years. It wouldn't have been healthy or responsible of me to remain in this strange woman's toxic presence.

I almost made it to the door when she yelled something about me being ungrateful. She must have immediately called my mother because when I returned home, I was greeted by her shouting, "Because of the way you treated my attorney, I now have proof that you aren't right in the head! I'm putting the house on the market to get as far away from you as I can. And because you're mentally unstable, you're going on disability."

I said nothing before I walked to the nearest bathroom and threw up. I was in bed for two days with a migraine. My mind couldn't stop wrestling with the realization that these two women had been scheming behind my back and planning my future, believing that they had this right.

Did my mother know that in the future the radiation damage would get so bad that I would need the government's help? Why hadn't she ever discussed this with me? Why had she hired an attorney? What else didn't I know that my mother and her lawyer knew? Was I going to need to be institutionalized?

I didn't know what disability was back then, other than it was for people with disabilities. Was my mother's plan to let the government be responsible for me as I slowly declined into a vegetative state?

Artists have vivid imaginations and mine took off. My head felt like it was going to explode. My neck, spine, sacrum, and feet all hurt. My mother knew that stress affected me, and she used this to get her revenge for what I supposedly did to her.

Was she trying to increase the migraines and intentionally weaken me, so the government would have to help? Could the attorney obtain my health records without my consent?

But I'm a grown woman! I have rights—though not according to my mother or her lawyer. They acted like they had the right to force me to do whatever they wanted. They didn't care that I'd been working diligently for years to get myself better, and that I had plans of my own.

Having a migraine scrambles your brain. But I really had to think.

Could this attorney have me declared incompetent? What was the point of just sitting and glaring at me? And why did she want to compare migraines, which only made her look really stupid? I knew that Gainor wouldn't hesitate to tell me if something was wrong. I could trust her and Lori, too. They'd both confirm that I was not crazy. They'd both stick up for me.

Being with Lori the next day in her office that exuded a warm and comforting welcome, I finally felt safe again.

"I'm not just feeling angry about these two women trying to take control of my life. After all these years that I've been sick, I've finally reached my limit. I'm reassessing everything. The two medications I took ruined my life, and they accomplished nothing. I'm done, Lori."

I got a lump in my throat and had to pause to compose myself. "If I hadn't taken them, I never would have had to live with my mother and discover how ugly she and my two siblings can be. And my career had been about to take off."

Lori sat silently, looking sympathetic.

"How is it even possible for my mother and siblings and this whacky lawyer to not know or care that there are two perspectives in every relationship? All that seems to matter to them is what they think. How can they be so shallow?"

"Under stress, people tend to think in narrow-minded ways," Lori said with a soft gentleness.

"If I can think more expansively with the stress I'm under, is it too much to ask this of others?"

"I don't think you're giving yourself enough credit."

"The migraines keep increasing in strength and frequency and I'm scared, Lori. I have done my best to treat my mother with love and patience, but she's creating this absurd grand finale before she leaves, about me being a liar and saying I'm not right in my head."

I leaned my body forward and placed my elbows on my knees, and covered my face with both hands. After a moment I sat up and said, "Something I've never even told you, Lori. After I was on *20/20*, they called wanting to do a follow-up show."

I paused to stop myself from crying. "Can you imagine how this would have affected my career? I wasn't home and my mother answered the phone. Instead of taking a message like most people do, she yelled into the phone, 'My daughter's dying!'" I stopped and felt the pain of this to help it pass right through me and finally leave my body.

"I don't know if she purposely sabotaged me or was just being her overly dramatic self. Or both. Either way, they're no longer interested."

I took a moment to compose myself. "And you know what? I didn't get angry at her when she told me this. I never told her that she destroyed my big chance. This was something I had worked for years to create. Despite what my siblings think, I have never intentionally hurt my mother. Maybe if I did, I wouldn't get as many migraines and I'd get better sooner, but I would never be able to live with myself."

***

About a week later, without any warning, my mother said, "Get out."

I lived in my studio for almost a month with my cat, Buster, who ran around at night trying to catch bats as they flew overhead. Consequently, I didn't get much sleep.

"Of course, you're upset with your mother," Gainor said. "Who the hell told you you're not allowed to be? Are you aware of how often you defend your mother and siblings? Yet you're always apologizing for yourself. You're too nice and they take advantage of you."

I have to set stronger boundaries.

"You think losing Groton Long Point—your childhood home—shouldn't have an effect on you? In your fragile and vulnerable state? Give me a break."

"My mother has been talking about selling her house for years. But she never had the courage. Yelling at the hospital about selling it gave her the perfect excuse to move. When I told her that the hospital and doctors weren't going to charge me and I didn't need her to sell her house, she actually got upset with me."

"If your mother really cared about you, why wouldn't she have asked me or Lori what we thought before doing this? If I didn't know better, I'd swear your mother was an alcoholic."

Gainor had been an active member of AA for over 25 years at this time and yet, even after she said this, I didn't take it seriously. My mother hardly drank at all.

Losing Groton Long Point took the air out of my sails. It had given me a foundation, a consistency, a sense of freedom, openness, nurturing, and a feeling of unlimited possibilities since I was young.

I had always spent my summers fishing as a kid, sitting on East Dock with my feet dangling, and waving to boaters as they passed by. When I wasn't fishing, I was either crabbing or collecting mussels that hung from the rocks that framed the peninsula's three-mile shoreline. I used to leap from one large boulder to another while trying to soar high in the air, feeling completely free.

It wasn't easy rebuilding my life as a 47-year-old single woman with a degree in Fine Arts who kept getting exhausted from what I called full body migraines. Losing Groton Long Point felt like a death to me. I still grieve this loss.

After I moved into my new home, I got the longest and most painful migraine I'd ever had. It forced me into bed for ten long, miserable days.

It was only because a friend had given me a water cooler that I had placed by my bedside months before that water was accessible, and I didn't die because I wasn't strong enough to stand and drink water from the nearest sink. This was before cell phones, and I was too weak to walk to the kitchen to use the phone to call for help. I had to crawl to use the bathroom, stopping often to rest. Because I didn't have the energy to crawl back into bed, I often slept on the bathroom floor.

I thought perhaps my body was telling me I should have died a long time ago, and this was the price I had to pay because I didn't. I wanted to die. I didn't want to kill myself. I just wanted the pain to end.

***

Standing for long periods of time—such as in the shower—used to be too tiring, so for years I'd only taken baths. After living in my new home for a while, I was finally able to take a shower. I was feeling happy and grateful to have this fragment of normalcy back. This is probably what helped me connect the dots because suddenly I knew why my mother had changed.

With the warm water streaming over me, I realized my mother had a drug addiction. The more I thought about it, the more convinced I was. The extreme change in her behavior pointed in this direction: She had total disregard for any harm she caused. She had become aggressive and verbally violent and often shown delusional behavior. She had become far more irritable, argumentative, and defensive than she had ever been. She was in complete denial, often rationalizing, offering excuses and justifications for her often-inexplicable behavior. She got easily confused and would try to hide it by using diversion tactics such as changing the subject to cover her befuddlement or becoming accusatory. As the shower's warm water comforted me, I thought about our last conversation.

"Mom, I'm just calling to say I love you. How are you? Are you still going to acupuncture and swimming in the pool?"

"It rained and there are large pools of water in front of my condo, so I have to be careful when I go out, so my feet don't get wet."

"I meant swimming in the pool like you do for exercise."

"I know what you meant, Sandi. You do this all the time to me. I'm just saying I can't go swimming because it's raining. I miss the weather in Connecticut. I wish I'd never sold my house."

The more I thought about it, the more her being addicted made perfect sense. Taking drugs was something she always did to avoid her problems. For weeks, I fought against believing this, but I knew in my heart that it was true. After wrestling with this sickening thought, I called my brother to share my thoughts.

"If I had all the problems Mom has, I would have a so-called drug addiction, too," he said, resisting facing this possibility even more than I did.

Our sister lived only ten minutes from our mother and she had never said anything about Mom's drug use, so I thought maybe I could be wrong, not really wanting to be right. Since my siblings weren't on the same page with me, there was nothing I could do about it anyway.

My sister drove my mother to her doctor's appointments. Long after I began suspecting my mother had an addiction, a doctor told my sister our mother was taking more drugs than any of his other patients, to which my sister replied that our mother got prescriptions from other doctors, too. This was how her addiction to opioids got exposed.

Pharmaceutical companies had assured the medical world that opioids weren't addictive. For years, doctors prescribed them without giving it a second thought. By the 1990s, the use of opioids for chronic pain had considerably increased. This was most likely when my mother got hooked. The United States Department of Health and Human Services declared opioids a public health emergency in 2017, but for my mother, and my siblings and me, this was much too late.

My sister now called me often because our mother was making her life unbearable. I would listen and offer my support, though I was hoping she would realize that I lived for years *with* our addicted mother and *while* I was sick and struggling. And Mom was telling lies about me and I had no idea why. But my sister was really struggling so I did my best to support her.

Patiently I waited for my sister to appreciate that I had lived with the horrors of our mother's addiction without all the advantages that she had.

I told her I thought Mom got addicted after her third husband died but my sister thought it was earlier, and perhaps it was. The point that I was trying to make is that Mom was addicted during the years that I lived with her. But when I came right out and said this, my sister changed the subject. She only wanted to talk about her own problems.

Shortly after I had moved in with my mother, she acted surprised when I told her I knew she had used drugs after I got the brain tumor. This may be why my mother viewed me as a threat from this moment on. To keep her addiction from being exposed, she told lies about me—quintessential behavior for a drug addict.

There was a side of me that felt better once I knew my mother had been addicted to opioids when I lived with her. At least I understood what had destroyed our relationship, especially after I read that drugs affect our brain's prefrontal cortex, which is responsible for rational thinking and decision-making. And that with misuse, drugs give someone a distorted view of reality and make it difficult to think beyond their own immediate need to use.

Thomas Harrison and Hillary Connery wrote in their book, *The Complete Family Guide to Addiction*, "For both addicts and their families, it's the world's most bewildering, maddening, and frightening illness." I can certainly attest to that.

After finding herself sandwiched between providing a home for me and keeping her addiction hidden, my mother created an ingenious plan. She convinced both my siblings, who knew she loved drama and often made up things, that I had been abusing her. She gained the attention of all three of her children in a way she had never had before. And she fought hard to hold on to this victorious position. She wasn't about to give up having this spotlight on her and go back to being the lonely, depressed widow she was before I moved in with her.

Even if this did break my heart and ostracize me from my family, and made getting radiation damage more brutal, even if I was diagnosed with having PTSD from this and all that I'd been through, I still think my mother's scheme was quite impressive. This was not an easy plan to devise, orchestrate, and implement. It showed how creative and intelligent—and desperate—a woman my mother was. She hid her addiction from all three of her children for at least 10 years while gaining my siblings' attention and blind loyalty.

When People Show Their Discontent

Long after I became an adult, I continued to only want to see the good in people. Even after someone wasn't kind to me, I chalked it up to them as having a bad day. After I got sick, I saw that most people were loving and supportive and wanted me to be happy and succeed. But there were a few people who hadn't yet learned how to be happy and fulfill their hearts. Because they couldn't, they tried to hurt me in a myriad of ways.

Particularly when vulnerable, you need to protect yourself from harm. List the ways you have successfully avoided allowing other people to hurt you.

_____

_____

_____

_____

_____

_____

_____

Keep a list of the times someone hurt you, what you did, and what you might do to avoid being hurt in the future. What did this cost you, and how might you better respond to hurtful people?

_____

_____

_____

_____

_____

_____

_____

18

We Aren't Meant to Be Strong All the Time

I was enjoying the afterglow and the scent of lavender that permeated the air after a Reiki session. When the session was over, I opened my eyes and saw Ellie, the practitioner, crying as she tried to compose herself.

She apologized and explained, "I know this is very unprofessional of me, but I know who you are. I mean, I don't really know you because we've never met, but years ago, I saw your mural, right after my mother died. While I was there and feeling the love you somehow painted into it, I felt my mother's love again."

It was still touching people's hearts this deeply after all these years? All I could do was smile in gratitude and touch my open hand to my heart.

"I read about your story in the local newspapers, and saw you on TV," said Ellie. "Even before I saw it, I knew you painted it from your heart."

What a gift this is to be hearing this.

"When I walked into the gallery, I was so surprised to feel my mother's love. I now have proof that my mother never really died, and her love and spirit will always be with me."

"Thank you for this gift you're giving *me*," I said.

"You gave me back a part of my life I thought I lost forever," she continued. "You've changed so many people's lives and you probably don't even know what you've done because sharing your love is natural to you."

"I really am deeply touched by what you're saying."

"When I was giving you a Reiki session, my mother's love came through you again. Your heart is so open that her love flows through you."

"To help heal myself, I kept my heart open as much as I could and still do." I sat up from the table, opened my arms, and the two of us hugged in appreciation of each other. "I feel privileged to be able to share your mother's love with you. I came here today for an additional boost of energy, and I sure got it. The heck with professionalism. I'll take sharing love any day," I said.

"Would you mind telling me more about how you used love to help you heal?" Ellie asked.

"I suspect you've figured a lot of this out yourself, but as I see it, when we take good care of ourselves and treat ourselves lovingly, we can share love with each other far more easily," I said. "I think love connects us with our Source, because God, or whatever you choose to call this, is the highest form of love there is."

"Yes. I believe that, too."

"When we overcome our own personal barriers," I said, "by keeping ourselves grounded and our hearts open, we remove the walls that block us, so we can share, receive, and feel love more freely. We just have to remember that love is always available."

"So often life gets in our way and distracts us. That's my biggest challenge."

"Mine, too," I said. "I think we all get challenged by everyday life. I still have to keep reminding myself to let every situation be what it is, instead of what I want it to be. Whenever someone triggers me, I use this annoyance as a reminder to work on my own issues."

"That's a great way to use our resistance, so we don't close ourselves off to love," Ellie said.

"When we can accept how someone acts because of his life experiences, we can feel compassion for him, instead of annoyance. But it's clear to me that you already know a lot about this because of all the work that you have done."

***

In December 2009, I was diagnosed with breast cancer, another one of the many side effects from the radiation damage that had been tormenting my life for the last 15 years. Most people know that supporting oneself as an artist isn't easy. Getting breast cancer devastated me on many levels.

I was still getting migraines, often multiple times each week. And before I would fully recuperate, another one erupted. Since they interfered with my ability to work, I was struggling financially. Because a large percentage of my earnings was spent on my health care, after I got breast cancer, I didn't know how I would support myself.

"The diagnosis of breast cancer can send your mind spinning in a hundred different directions. Right after diagnosis, being in panic mode is normal," wrote Dr. Veronique Desaulniers, who had worked in the wellness field since 1979 and was a breast cancer survivor herself.

Panicking was exactly how I reacted, in a way that was far different from when I was told I had the brain tumor and would soon die.

In the words of Dr. Desaulniers, "Breast cancer is probably one of the most feared diagnoses a woman can get. The mere mention of it conjures up images of death, despair, or at best, disfigurement."

When my doctor called to tell me I had breast cancer, I was alone, volunteering at the Westerly Cooperative Art Gallery. It was December, the best selling time of the year. I didn't want to keep my fellow artists from selling their art just because I had gotten bad news, so I stayed until my shift ended and then rushed home. Before I even removed my coat, I called my sister to tell her. As our mother's addiction had grown worse, we had been talking almost every day.

I was under the impression that my sister appreciated my forgiving her for how she had treated me in the past. I thought she was grateful for all the support I had been giving her as she struggled with the changes in our mother. To show her how much I loved and trusted her, and to demonstrate that I truly had forgiven her, I told her that she would be the first person I called after I got my biopsy results.

The first thing I said to her before I even said hello was, "I have breast cancer." After holding this in for hours and finally releasing it, I got dizzy and light-headed. To my surprise, my sister said something. What? That she would call me back?

"But I have cancer," I shouted, scared to be alone in my diminishing state. But the only thing I heard was nothingness.

Thirteen years before, when I told Gary I had a brain tumor, he was unable to support me. When my doctors told me I had radiation damage and part of the AVM could once again be life-threatening, my mother could only scream in fear. When I called my biological father to ask questions about his mother who had died of a brain tumor, his emotions must have gotten the best of him because he gasped after about a minute, hung up the phone, and never called me back.

To avoid feeling obliterated like this again, to make sure I got the support I needed this time, I gave my sister time to prepare herself by telling her the day before that I would be calling after I heard from my doctor. She knew how she had treated me in the past. I was giving her this opportunity to make up for this. Didn't most people know not to put their sister on hold after she said she had cancer?

Being treated again as if I had no value, being pushed aside and having my feelings not considered, being left on my own like this because another person put their own needs first again, was beyond my capabilities. I held my phone to my ear, believing I would hear my sister's voice again, that she had to be there, that she wouldn't leave me knowing I just said I had cancer. She knew that I lived alone. And yet somehow, she had forgotten to ask if I was alright before she hung up the phone.

For the first time in my life, I fell apart. I broke down in a way I didn't recognize. I must have gone into shock, fainted or something, because all I remembered was entering some strange foreign place that had a hazy, airy-like and foggy atmosphere where everything moved in slow motion. It felt like I was falling in a slow, topsy-turvy way into a cold godless space, like I was disappearing into some black hole, and I was never going to be able to come back again. Perhaps I had reached my limit and something inside me actually did die.

I don't know how much time passed. It was the feeling of the cold tile floor on the side of my face that brought me back into this world. I was crying when I woke up, but I didn't know why. I couldn't remember what happened until I saw my phone on the floor.

My first thought was to call 911, but I didn't know what I would say when the dispatcher answered. All I knew was I didn't feel safe, that I was scared, and everything felt hazy, and it was hard to think. Something about my sister? And I had cancer?

The phone rang, and I jumped. Frightened and confused, I let it ring a few times before I answered it. The person at the other end of the line claimed to be my sister. I listened to the voice, believing this had to be someone impersonating her. My sister wouldn't be so cruel as to hang up on me, thinking she could just call me back at her convenience.

I was too frightened to talk. I was afraid that whatever I told this person on the phone would be used against me. I had to protect myself because I couldn't afford to be hurt again in the vulnerable state that I was in. The voice sounded like my sister, and asked me how I was. Afraid to answer her question, I told her I didn't know.

"You're probably feeling vulnerable," the voice said.

Oh no! She knew! This couldn't be good. I didn't say much. I let the voice do the talking.

I don't know why my sister stopped talking to me on this day, because no matter how often I asked, she refused to tell me what she thought I did wrong.

Years later, when I shared with my therapist how out-of-it I'd become and how hazy everything had gotten, Alexis assured me that how I responded was the quintessential way a traumatized person would act. She told me that passing out, the hole I fell into, and the days I spent in bed afterwards, feeling paranoid and afraid of the world, were normal reactions to be expected. She assured me I hadn't been damaged beyond repair, and I could learn to trust again with work and time.

The PTSD I'd thought was long behind me reared its ugly head and wouldn't let go of me for years to come. I'd loudly scream if someone surprised me. Hardly a day would pass when I didn't cry. Trusting others became a serious problem. I also lost my desire to socialize.

***

Why would anyone stop talking to her sister on the day she was told she had breast cancer? I asked myself for months, trying to understand my sister's actions. And I asked my friends too.

Carrying this heavy emotional weight around, while trying to overcome breast cancer, angered and inflamed the migraines. They surged with a vengeance. I needed to find a way to make peace with my sister's decision or I was going to be in even bigger trouble. Something in me clicked when a friend said, "Your sister sounds so emotionally imbalanced that she has to withdraw. There's no way she can consider you. I'm guessing she's ignoring you, just like she ignores her own problems."

I said, "What you said makes so much sense, but it makes me feel sick. I hate thinking of my sister being this damaged.

"Particularly because you have cancer, you've got to remember how your sister is acting has nothing to do with you. Your mother uses drugs, and your brother screams and has to put others down to make himself feel good. But the worst thing is that everyone in your family refuses to look at themselves and learn from their mistakes."

"I really do feel nauseous because I know you're right."

***

I had survived a life-threatening brain tumor, coped with the endless symptoms from radiation damage, including breast cancer. I had lived with two angry and aggressive drug addicts who had blamed me for their problems for years. I used to get panic attacks. For decades, I'd coped with excruciating migraines that left me so exhausted I got chronic fatigue syndrome. I had been fine-tuning my body, doing all I could so I remained physically and emotionally balanced to help me heal, but the migraines still continued to disrupt my life.

Because of my financial pressures, the migraines and my sadness, and the continual struggles from the radiation symptoms, by the time I was diagnosed with breast cancer, I didn't know if I could fight it. Or if I wanted to, or if I even had the right to expect anything more from my battered body. I wondered, since I was supposed to die decades ago, if I should just appreciate how strong my body has been and be grateful for the time I've been given.

Knowing I would be upsetting my family again, as my sister's reaction confirmed, I considered letting the cancer just run its course. Long ago my family had made it clear that they'd reached their limit, so wasn't it understandable that I'd finally reached mine?

I had worked so hard to forgive and befriend my sister, and put in so much time and effort nurturing our relationship. I'd supported her for so long, listening practically every day to the problems she had with our mother, only to have her exit from my life in such a brutal way when I needed her.

When she got married decades before, she chose me to be her maid of honor. And if anything were to happen to her and her husband, it was me she chose to bring up her children. So, what happened?

This was too unhealthy. I couldn't take it anymore. Something had to change. And I had to change it. In an attempt to put an end to this, I chose to concentrate on how much I loved my sister.

Even if I couldn't ever trust her ever again, I knew I could trust the love I felt for her. Rather than continuing to torture myself by yearning for her love and acceptance, every time I felt this, I stopped and sent her love. This created space that allowed me to experience the love I thought I'd lost. It opened doors that freed me from this pain's tight grip. Eventually, I felt grateful that I had a sister that I could love.

***

After being diagnosed with cancer, I reached out to my friends for help and got a support team who understood me better than I did myself. Every time I expressed how ashamed and guilty I felt for becoming emotionally disjointed, each of these dear women assured me that how I acted was to be expected. That I wasn't being a troublemaker, or a pain in the butt, as I believed.

These women told me they wanted to help; that they weren't secretly feeling resentful of me. From them, I learned I had to not only face my pain and grief, but again that I had to accept my family's behavior or it was going to continue to devour me.

"I should be used to how my family acts by this time," I kept saying, believing I was somehow wrong for having such a difficult time accepting how cruel they could be.

It felt foreign to be treated with this much love and understanding. In the past, when I had been sick and living with my mother or Gary, I was never treated so lovingly.

"All you did was get breast cancer. You've done nothing wrong, not to your family or anyone, so please stop feeling so guilty. You know how good it feels to help others, so hear me when I say I sincerely want to help you, Sandi," my friend Julianne told me.

Several people recommended a local naturopath who specialized in cancer. This doctor told me I ought to consider myself lucky to have the kind of cancer that could be cut from my body. She suggested I go home and schedule the lumpectomy and put this all behind me.

Frightened and befuddled, and not at my strongest, I followed her advice because I believed a naturopathic physician would tell me if cancer could be treated naturally, since this is what I told her I was looking for.

After I had two lumpectomies, my surgeon said that I was now to have six weeks of radiation to decrease my chances of the cancer returning by just seven percent. And I had to take Tamoxifen. But I had gotten radiation decades before and I still suffered from the side effects. I felt ambushed and surprised to only be hearing this now —after I had the two surgeries. I cried and declined further treatment.

"Ms. Gold, it would be unfair to not tell you that you are making a poor choice," this surgeon said. "Don't take this the wrong way, but I think you definitely could use a good therapist."

A year later, the cancer returned. When I was told I had to have a mastectomy, I declined this, too.

Feeling Compassion for Others

According to Psychology Today, *"Compassion is an empathetic understanding of a person's feelings, accompanied by altruism, or a desire to act on that person's behalf." When you can accept that people act like they do because of their life experiences, it's easier to feel compassion even when someone hurts you. If a person's tendency is to treat others poorly, imagine what their life must be like. I found compassion to be a powerful tool—as long as I didn't take it too far. Just because someone hurt me and I felt compassion for them, didn't mean my being hurt didn't matter.*

The next time someone hurts you, remember that this is because of their past. Can you both address your hurt and have compassion for them?

Write down the times you didn't successfully accomplish this. How might you have better protected yourself and what did this cost you because you didn't?

_____

_____

_____

_____

_____

_____

_____

_____

_____

_____

_____

_____

_____

_____

_____

_____

19

Trust Your Intuition

Before I was diagnosed with cancer, unable to cope with the pain the migraines caused, I got a prescription for Imitrex. Though not a magic bullet, it did stop the pain, but it also left me with dizziness and fatigue. Plus, Imitrex was expensive.

Until I got this medication through a state patient assistance program for low-income people, I paid $20 for each pill I took, sometimes taking two or more pills per week for over two years.

Once I signed up for the program, I also received a free annual mammogram, and should I ever get breast cancer, all my expenses would be paid. Therefore, the two lumpectomies I had were covered by the state. However, when the cancer returned, and I declined a mastectomy and chose to use a natural protocol (that I was willing to pay for), I was dropped from this program.

Despite making a decision that would have saved the state thousands of dollars, there was no acknowledgement that there was more than just one treatment for everyone. Once again, I did not fit into the one-size-fits-all medical regimen.

***

In 2015, when former President Jimmy Carter announced that his melanoma had spread to his liver and brain, I, like many others, thought he would die. But he chose a treatment that combined radiation with immunotherapy, which uses the power of the immune system to prevent, control, and eliminate cancer. Conventional medicine was slowly catching up, working with our immune systems with remarkable success. Thankfully, it saved Jimmy Carter's life.

Four years before this, I beat the breast cancer by strengthening my immune system too, but I got booted from the state's assistance program. And because I chose a natural treatment, they also dropped my health insurance. I called Dr. Lillian Poston, a retired nurse and kinesiologist (among many other specialties), who had been offering me her services at no cost for years. I told her my doctors said I had to get a mastectomy. She met me at the door of her home with a warm and loving smile.

"I think you already know what you need to do. You've become quite skilled at listening to your body. I have faith that you'll find what you are looking for and you'll be just fine. May I get you some tea?"

Over a decade before, Lori had suggested I see this woman. "I can't explain what she does, but she's a brilliant, multi-talented, lovely woman. Even allopathic doctors respect her. One even calls her a human MRI."

Shortly after I scheduled my first appointment with Dr. Lillian, I received an envelope in the mail from her. As I pulled her numerous brochures out, small plastic gold angels flew from the envelope and into the air, making me laugh out loud.

I was on steroids at this time and couldn't drive. A friend drove me to my first appointment. When he pulled his car up to her house, both of us sat there speechless. Over a small flower garden loomed a large, wooden, handmade archway that framed her front door. Colorful banners reading "love" and "peace" were flapping about in the wind. Statues of angels in various sizes and shades of gray stood intermingled among the multicolored flowers.

I grinned in delight. The plan had been that my friend would wait in his car for me and read his book, so I was confused when he opened his car door when I opened mine.

"I'm going in with you," he whispered. "This woman could be a witch."

Years later, I shared this story with Dr. Lillian. "Please assure your friend that this isn't the first time someone has thought this," she said and giggled.

Though only 4'11", she had a huge and regal presence. When she walked into a room, one couldn't help noticing that she glowed with love and joy. Soon after meeting her, she became my mentor.

One of the many things she helped me understand, years before I knocked on her door with breast cancer, is why one day, while working on my computer, I suddenly collapsed and fell into it after hearing on NPR that Senator Tim Johnson's AVM had burst. Until Dr. Lillian explained why, I had no idea what made my body react like it did. And I'd lived in fear of it happening again.

She explained that my buried fears (of the AVM bursting and killing me) had grown over the years and would only surface when I felt safe enough to feel this amount of fear and horror. She thought it was a good thing that my body had collapsed. She even danced around the room and shouted "Yahoo!" with her arms waving high above her head. She smiled and congratulated me for creating a safe environment that allowed me to feel the intensity of this fear that I had been carrying in my body for years.

I asked, "Do you remember what you said after I told you I was glad I was alone in my studio when I collapsed because I would have terrified anyone who saw this? You told me that I go out of my way not to upset others and I often act in a way that's detrimental to myself for the sake of others' comfort."

"Yes. I have seen you make this sacrifice often."

"I thought about this a lot and why I keep doing this. Probably because I grew up believing my job was to help my mother in every way I could, because she always encouraged this. I grew up believing that love meant putting others' needs first."

"It's wonderful that you have such a loving heart. The problem is when you put others' needs before your own, you unknowingly sacrifice yourself and your health."

"The very first time I needed my family's help, they turned against me like an angry mob. I still feel badly because this really scared and angered me."

"Letting your anger rip the way you did was a healthy thing. I would hate to see the shape your body would be in today if it hadn't known it *had* to vent. Like pressure cookers, people need to blow when there's too much pressure put on them."

"I can't believe you just said that! That's exactly what I needed to hear. You just gave me the additional strength I need to fight this breast cancer."

"I'm sorry your family didn't understand this. That they thought you should always put their needs first, even when you were so sick. Do you think you'll ever be able to forgive yourself for responding in the natural and healthy way you did? Your body needs you to understand that you acted like you did in order to survive."

"I was weighed down by guilt for many decades because I had a temper—even though I knew the tumor caused it. I even had to sleep on a frozen cold pack for years because my head got so hot when I laid it on my pillow. I literally had a hot head. Thank you for explaining all this."

I confessed to Dr. Lillian that I used to feel guilty about the agony my family experienced. Because I was in so much pain while I was living with my mother, two or three times, when I was driving and another car in the other lane was coming in my direction, it felt like my steering wheel was being pulled from my hands. Like it was being turned in the direction of the oncoming car. Before this happened to me, I always thought that people chose to commit suicide. That it wasn't some kind of pulling sensation that occurred that caused their death.

"It was only because I didn't want to hurt the other driver that I didn't drive head on into them."

"So again, you used love to help you. This is you, Sandi. Celebrate this!"
"Awwww. Thanks."

"I also want to tell you that it's a good thing you weren't driving when your body collapsed and you fell into your computer. If you had been, we probably wouldn't be having this conversation. You do realize you could have been killed, which just proves how serious ignoring your feelings and refusing to feel them is."

"I have never thought about it like this before."

"This is why you must surround yourself with people who listen, respect, and want to help you, not humiliate, shame you, and make things harder. Only share yourself with people who have the ability to appreciate you."

Meaning never seeing my family again?

"You're an artist, and artists need to express themselves. Only allow people into your life who are willing to face their demons, like you do. People who have no need to blame and find fault with you just because *they're* struggling emotionally. They have no right to demand that you do this for them just because they're not willing to do it for themselves."

This is exactly what my family does.

"Surround yourself with people who feel honored to listen and learn from you. You do know that I've learned from you, too? We all learn from each other. It's essential that we listen with open hearts and respect one another, but remember, not everyone does this."

People who let fear guide them. And not love.

"Would you please allow me to suggest that you recognize all you've achieved? Someday you'll look back and see having breast cancer as just a blip on the screen. You've got this, Sandi. You really do."

We Are All Individuals

Why would anyone think everyone is supposed to think like they do? Is it because when people think differently than they do, this creates too much discomfort? And their comfort is their only interest? Our experiences shape the way we act and think, so expecting someone to think like they do is not healthy for anyone. Every person deserves the right to live and think how they choose. Write down the number of times you tried to control someone. In what ways might you break this habit and be more respectful of others?

Keep a list of the times someone tried to control you. How did this feel?

_____

_____

_____

_____

_____

_____

_____

_____

Did you like this exercise? How did you handle this?

_____

_____

_____

_____

_____

_____

_____

_____

20

You Must Learn Your Body's Language

I had never heard of anyone overcoming cancer using natural means. My biggest challenge was finding a natural treatment. I told as many people as I could what I was looking for and did my own research. Less than two weeks later, my friend BJ handed me a copy of Bill Henderson's protocol and said, "You might want to consider this."

Every cell in my body responded with a definite *yes!*

When I was about six or seven, my mother joined the Milford Yacht Club. Rather than enjoy all the amenities it offered like the rest of my family did, I used to walk down to the town's public pier just minutes away, where I would fish for hours.

We moved to Groton Long Point when my mother remarried, and I was still in elementary school. Here I spent summers fishing off East Dock, just two blocks from my home. This felt like heaven. Gazing over the Fishers Island Sound with my fishing rod in my hand, I decided that God wouldn't have created mankind as impressively as He had and leave us all defenseless. I later learned in my science class that our bodies had immune systems.

"I knew it. I just knew it," I smugly thought.

I was riding in the backseat of my family's light blue Ford station wagon on the way to Long Island to spend Thanksgiving with relatives when I was about 13. Though I enjoyed seeing my cousins, I hated this four-hour-long, heavily-trafficked trip. As we approached the outskirts of New York City, I used to stare out the window gaping at the poverty in disbelief, saddened that there were people who lived like this. Being highly sensitive to smells, I was repulsed by an offensive chemical odor that invaded our car as we drove by one particular area.

I had been spoiled waking up to the smell of saltwater and the sounds of seagulls crying overhead as they dropped clams on our black shingled roof, while preparing their fresh seafood breakfast. I especially loved waking up on foggy mornings. I'd pull my covers up to my chin and keep my eyes closed while I listened to the nurturing sound of the North Dumpling foghorn. Its low, sluggish bass sound punctured through the morning silence and traveled across the water to my appreciative ears.

When I caught the first whiff of this chemical smell, I would hold my breath for as long as I could. When I absolutely had to breathe again and was forced to inhale this foul toxin, I hoped that my and my family's immune systems were doing their jobs. As the road separated us from this least favorite leg of our trip, I prayed that these fumes weren't cancerous, and none of our lives had just been cut short.

I was 58 years old when I was told that the cancer had spread and I had to get a mastectomy. I had just read that our ability to heal is significantly increased when we have family support. I knew how my family would respond when they heard I had this second round of cancer.

I decided it wasn't fair of me to doubt my body's capabilities. My body had always been faithful to me, even if my family hadn't. It had been working on my behalf all my life and had already proven its amazing abilities. Now, it was my turn to assist it, and show my love and loyalty.

If I made the wrong decision, my doctor said this could cost me my life. But I had outlived five doctor's wrong predictions before and done the impossible more than once. I had more faith in my body than I did in any doctor. Plus, if I died, no one in my family would probably care. And maybe by choosing to use a natural treatment, I would be helping advance medicine.

"I'm not going to die," I told myself because cancer was no match for us—meaning to God, my Creator, my body, and me. What better way was there to honor and show my love and appreciation for the life I had been given?

Though I wouldn't suggest this to anyone, I overcame breast cancer by strengthening my immune system without the help of a doctor. I had no money or health insurance at this time. I had been teaching myself ways to manage stress for decades by this time. I had become quite proficient at understanding my body, being attuned to what it was saying, and trusting, and following its unfailing love and loyalty. And I trusted love to guide me.

By staying focused and strengthening myself in whatever ways I could, despite still getting migraines, lacking in finances, and without my family's emotional or any doctor's support, I succeeded in overcoming more than just breast cancer. I learned to trust the way the world was created.

I was fortunate I hadn't waited until I had breast cancer before I understood my body's language and made a habit of addressing whatever triggered me. And I knew that stress affects our bodies and had already learned some ways to manage mine. Getting the brain tumor, radiation damage, and breast cancer had been an invaluable way to get to know myself, and how and why my body and I reacted in certain ways.

I first began to learn about my body's wisdom when I lived in Washington, D.C. from Dr. Lynn Brallier, but it was Lori who taught me to truly appreciate my body's remarkable abilities. She also helped me to know myself better. For years, I got to see myself through Lori's eyes, which gave me the tools and confidence to overcome anything, including the cancer I got years after I stopped seeing her.

"Be proud of yourself. No matter how painful things got, I never saw you hesitate to do the work," she told me at our last appointment. "Other people use avoidance tactics when things get tough, but you've always faced your demons head-on and willingly made the needed changes."

"But I was scared. I've got to admit there were times this was really frightening."

"But you had the courage and not everyone does. And you never once wavered from letting love guide you. Sure, there were times you got angry, but you had every right to be."

"I wasn't allowed to get angry when I was a kid and not even after I got the brain tumor. I wasn't allowed to express my frustrations in front of Gary or my family."

"You'll probably find that the same people who criticized you will be envious and want what you have. They'll have no idea of the amount of pain you've endured or how much time you've invested. Your family has a habit of blaming others, but have you noticed that blaming is something you never do?"

"Blaming takes away our strength and power. I can't afford this."

"You buckle down and resolve problems. Have you ever wondered how long the brain tumor began to affect your life before it was diagnosed? Since you were born with it, I'm guessing that you found ways to cope with how it was affecting you as a child without even realizing this."

"As a kid, I tried so hard to be good, Lori. But every once in a while, I got really upset and lost it. I'd run to my room, slam the door, and throw all the shoes in my closet against it. I hated it when my mother, rather than listening to my frustrations, would spoon-feed me honey mixed with whiskey until I fell asleep."

"Good thing you didn't hold your feelings in like your siblings do, leaving you angry and resentful like them. Have you ever considered what might have happened if you hadn't gotten angry when you were little? I'm sorry that your siblings appear to not have the courage that you do, and they take their frustrations out on you."

"My childhood confused me. When my parents separated, I was only three or four. My father told me he would only be gone for two weeks. I was playing outside when he was packing his car. The young me looked into the trunk and saw our turquoise towels stacked in the upper right-hand corner."

"And your body told you something wasn't right?"

"I knew my father had lied. But what bewildered me even more over the next few weeks was that my mother and siblings acted as if everything was fine—because they all stuffed their feelings. I knew our life was changing. Yet, I questioned *myself* because no one else was acting sad."

"Your life has been altered in so many ways—your career, financially, and practically all of your relationships. You've been forced to make huge sacrifices, but you never grew bitter about this. Why do you think this is?"

"Because I refuse to live that way."

"Keeping up with the speed at which you're growing is going to be hard for most people, so be prepared for friends to leave you who are unable or unwilling to grow with you."

The same people who aren't willing to look at themselves will blame me for conflicts in our relationship.

"I'm guessing that your family thinks you got too big for your britches, and that you got what you deserved, Little Miss Smarty Pants."

I laughed as Lori straightened her spine and shook her body side-to-side, mimicking my family saying this.

"But most people change when they get a serious illness," she continued. "This is to be expected, and if friends and family aren't willing to accept this, learn, and grow too, there are bound to be problems. There will always be more challenges, but you now have the tools to help yourself. You know to listen to your body."

"I appreciate all you've done for me and all the tools you taught me. I have found that some tools come from the strangest places. Before I got sick and long after John Lennon died, I had a dream of him singing, 'It Won't Be Long Now.'" John was smiling and winking at me while playing on stage with the other Beatles. *It won't be long before what?* I wondered when I woke up."

"What do you think it means?"

"After I got the brain tumor, I thought about this dream. I think it meant it won't be long before I understood the love and joy that comes when we're true to ourselves; when we make love our priority, just like John did. He could have done anything with his life, but he chose to share love with us through his music."

"I think you'll have no problem finding the tools you need wherever you go."

"I'm in a much better position, in a more loving place than before I got the brain tumor. I understand people better. I can see that some people, like my family and Gary, will do anything *not* to face their pain. That they refuse or maybe they just can't look at their behavior and this stops them from growing and being happy."

"You've learned how much easier life is when you see the ways you need to grow. When you listen to your body's wisdom. Some people haven't learned this yet and some never will. This is something we all must accept, as difficult and sad as this is," Lori said.

"People used to tell me I was the black sheep in my family when I was growing up. I resented this because I loved my family. But I now see that if I was like them and I refused to take responsibility for how I felt and acted, I'd probably be dead now, huh?"

A sadness swept over me because accepting how different I was from my family created a feeling of separation. I still didn't like feeling detached from them, alone, and family-less.

"I think I was always different from them," I continued. "As a young teenager, I caught a small fish and watched as it was flapping on the dock. Moments later, its purplish-pink gills were the only thing that moved. I studied that fish until it died."

"I can see you doing that. You have such a delightful curiosity that has served you well."

"I wondered what had been in its body that was now gone. What had left without me seeing it leave? Some kind of life force dispersed in the air, the young me decided. Some kind of energy that gives us all life."

"And you were just a young teenager? Do you understand why I've been suggesting you look at who you are?"

"Yes. I can now see that no one else in my family thinks like I do. Shortly after I left for college, I became a vegetarian because I knew what gave that fish life, gave me life, too."

Lori leaned forward to show her interest.

"After I got radiation damage and my body felt 100 years old, I used to stand at the beach and inhale this same invisible life force that made the waves rise, curl, and crash back down before merging with the water again. I'd be thinking that this was what was going to help me heal."

"You seem to have always been attuned to life's energy, felt love, and life's supportive power. Even when you were young, you saw yourself as part of a much bigger picture."

"Maybe this also explains why, when I was a kid, thunderstorms scared and excited me. As soon as the sky darkened and I could feel this heightened energy, I would pedal my bike home as fast as I could. Sometimes I got caught in a strong wind and heavy rain. I told myself that this would pass. That the sun always shines again."

Lori smiled and nodded with encouragement.

"Maybe this helped me see that our darkest and most frightening times are just part of life. And that they always pass. Maybe knowing this sparked my determination to live after I was told I would die soon. I never really thought about this before. Is this what you mean? Is this what you want me to know about myself?"

You Were Created to be You
Who Does and Doesn't Appreciate You?

Maybe because I was born an artist, I have always had a need to be myself. Because I lacked confidence, I wasn't always faithful to this. Having people like Lori and Dr. Lillian reflect back on the good things they saw in me both helped me and inspired me to tell others what I admire about them. This has brought me closer to the people who understand it's also my responsibility to tell them if they do something that's unhealthy and hurts me. Much like Dr. Lillian suggested, surround yourself with people who appreciate you, and are grateful for what they can learn from you, and what you contribute to their lives.

Write down who tells you the things they appreciate about you and to whom you can speak your truth.

_____

_____

_____

_____

_____

_____

Who is quick to criticize you? How have you successfully dealt with their criticism and in what ways might you do better in the future? And who might you consider seeing less because it's unhealthy and you don't feel safe, at least for now?

_____

_____

_____

_____

_____

_____

21

Always, Always, Always Stay True to Yourself

Only five months after I began Bill Henderson's protocol to overcome breast cancer, I got my test results: both the mammogram and MRI showed no signs of cancer. I couldn't wait to tell my oncologist so his other patients could learn from this. But at my next appointment, before he even said hello, with a disapproving scowl on his face, he asked why I hadn't gotten the mastectomy.

I smiled and asked, "You haven't seen my test results?"

He flipped through a manila folder he held in his hands until he found what he was looking for. Appearing uncomfortable and stuttering his words, he replied, "Tests make mistakes," to which I said, "So do doctors."

He tried to convince me that my most recent tests, the ones that showed no cancer, were not reliable. And yet for some unexplained reason, he trusted the first tests, that ones that had shown I had cancer. What I found particularly disconcerting was that he offered no explanation as to why he thought this, despite my asking for clarification.

I am expected to ignore the most recent tests and believe only the first tests are right, even though he said tests make mistakes? I am to have my right breast removed based on his beliefs? This makes no sense to me.

Using a scare tactic, this doctor tried to convince me that if I didn't have the mastectomy, it could cost me my life. But I had been down this road before. Ever since I was diagnosed with the brain tumor, 25 years before, I had noticed a lot of people, not just doctors, believed they knew everything there was to know. And they expected me to think like them and got angry if I didn't. But I am responsible for myself and choosing what is best for me, not my doctors or my brother, who has never stopped screaming at me to do what he wants.

I kept thinking our Creator made us all as individuals and it would go against His wishes not to be the person I was created to be, and to think the way that I think. From this moment on, if someone only thought about what he wanted and no interest was shown in understanding my perspective, sirens went off inside my body. If someone failed to include me in a conversation that we were having, I was no longer willing to have this discussion.

Once home, I called to cancel my next appointment and was put on hold. Moments later, the oncologist got on the phone and tried to convince me again to think like him, but he offered no additional information and never asked to hear my perspective. He thought strong-arming me would work?

"You're playing with fire," he told me.

Because I had navigated through the horrors in my past, I knew myself and my body. I politely thanked him for sharing his opinion and hung up the phone.

This oncologist had an excellent reputation. He was a likeable and charming man. A friend of mine loved him. My naturopathic doctor recommended him, though she did admit the choices in our area were limited.

The type of care this doctor offered may be what other people wanted and chose for themselves, but I had spent a long time being a patient. I had learned that I got the best care when my doctors worked *with* me. And they didn't just expect me to follow their beliefs. I only use patient-centered healthcare. I refuse to be treated like a number. After I got the brain tumor, had I gone along with my doctor's beliefs, I could have died, so respecting my beliefs and following my heart is particularly important to me.

Health care is a for-profit business. It would be naïve to expect doctors to tell us that other options were available to help us besides what they practiced, any more than we could expect a restaurant to tell us what another restaurant offered on their menu. It's our responsibility to find both the doctor and the type of care that best fits our individual bodies' needs.

If you are someone who believes that doctors never make mistakes and you agree with everything every doctor does and you think that your medical care isn't affected by profit, then let them take control of you.

This is not what I do.

Too many doctors tried to coerce me into doing what they wanted. They refused to acknowledge that I had a voice and a perspective that was important. Many acted as if they didn't know that their patients' bodies held wisdom within them, and yet if our bodies didn't know how to heal, doctors wouldn't even exist.

I see doctors as part of my team and myself as the captain. I hire them to *assist* my healing, not to take charge. I use my doctors' expertise and knowledge as valuable tools to assist me in making my decisions. And unless there is an emergency, I take my time. Regardless of what your doctor prefers, make important decisions once you're relaxed in the comfort of your home. Both my oncologist and surgeon treated me as though I was expected to do everything they told me right there and then. Sirens went off in my head to warn me of danger when my surgeon followed me to the receptionist's desk and stood beside me and waited to make sure I made my next appointment. Even as experienced as I was, I felt intimidated and wasn't sure what to do. I made the appointment, knowing I could cancel it once I got home.

When I went for a biopsy, I explained to my surgeon that I had not yet decided how I planned to treat the spreading of the cancer. His eyebrows shot up and his brown eyes widened. When he saw my unwavering "don't give me any hassle" stare, he looked down before he answered.

"I wouldn't be comfortable if you waited more than a month before having the operation because it would be too dangerous to wait any longer," he said.

This conversation took place in 2011, and I never had the mastectomy. And every test I've had ever since has shown no sign of cancer. I don't expect other people to think like me or to make the same choices that I made. I encourage everyone to decide for themselves what is best for them.

Perhaps because I'm a gardener, I think like one. I know how important good soil is and the influence it has on the vegetables I grow. To me, it made more sense to make the environment in my body uninviting to the cancer. By changing where the cancer grew, as opposed to having my right breast removed, the chances would be better that the cancer would die since the "soil" in my body wasn't conducive to its needs.

My way of thinking simply differed from that of my doctors. What made me feel the safest and brought the most comfort was important to me, but apparently, it wasn't to them. This didn't even seem to be considered. Thanks to Dr. Kjellberg's sensitivity, I had learned how I needed and deserved to be treated. I was unwilling to settle for less.

I believed cancer could be cured naturally through diet, exercise, and supplements. My faith was so strong I was willing to risk my life on it. I understood that not everyone believed this. After all, we weren't created to all think alike.

Thanks to my mother insisting on coming to the hospital with me and my acquiescing to her wishes, I had learned (the hard way) the importance of being true to myself. No longer would I make a decision according to anyone else's beliefs or desires. When I was diagnosed with cancer in 2009, it wasn't unusual to see bowls of candy in doctors' offices. There was also candy where a friend went for chemotherapy. Even back then, there was a wealth of information proving that sugar is harmful to people with cancer. So why was candy being offered to cancer patients? How was it possible for healthcare providers to not know how unhealthy this was?

After I got breast cancer, I paid even stricter attention to what was unhealthy and stressful to me. I continually made adjustments to my diet and lifestyle. Why didn't my oncologist suggest changing my unhealthy habits?

Having five neurologists tell me I would die 25 years earlier proved to be to my advantage because I knew, in a significant and unforgettable way, that doctors are not always right. We can't always trust what they tell us.

If I had not had the brain tumor and learned all that I did, I would have followed my doctors' advice and had the mastectomy. How could I not now wonder how many women have needlessly had this operation?

Naturally, there were moments when my confidence wavered. And I would shame myself for having these doubts. Today I believe questioning myself was a healthy thing because every time I felt unsure, my fears got me to think. This reinforced that I was doing what I wanted and was right for me.

Like high and low tides, it's also natural that we ebb and flow because we are human and aren't made of concrete. These uncomfortable moments when my doubts surfaced were not enjoyable. But we were created with feelings, and they are meant to be felt for a good reason. My discomfort allowed me to feel this, and because I didn't ignore or fight it, my conviction was strengthened.

I religiously followed the late Bill Henderson's book, *Cancer Free.* The first thing I did was change my diet. At first, I struggled and worried this was causing stress, compromising my immune system, and making it harder for my body to fight the cancer. I decided the healthiest and quickest way for this to change was to change myself. I focused on what I could eat, and not on what I couldn't. And I grew to love my new diet.

Because having cancer, or any life-threatening illness, often creates discomfort in others, it's not uncommon for people to tell us that we're not dealing with our sickness properly. At first, this puzzled me until I realized what they were saying was being said to make *them* more comfortable. But making a decision based on what brings other people's comfort is dangerous. It could even cost you your life.

Having discovered how vital our feelings are, and that I must not put others' comfort before my own, I began to allow myself to cry whenever my body wanted to cry: I was silently crying in a doctor's waiting room when a stranger sat down next to me and whispered, "I'm here for you if you need me."

This loving gesture was not only comforting, but it also reminded me to be true to myself and that I didn't always have to be strong. And that there would always be people who wanted to share their love with me.

***

Just months after I started the natural treatment, I had a frustrating setback, though not from another side-effect: My home got infested with fleas.

To most people, discovering a flea in their home is annoying. They might believe, as I did, that chemical bombs are the only way to get rid of them. But I had been using a natural treatment to overcome breast cancer, eating organic foods, using only natural products on my body, and making my own cleaning products. Chemicals create an environment inside our bodies where cancer flourishes.

When I felt a bloodthirsty flea bite my ankle, my heart pounded as I heard my oncologist's words, "If your cancer begins to grow again, it will with vengeance. If it spreads, you could die."

My most recent HCG test (a home test I took every eight weeks to test the amount of cancer in my body) had for the first time shown that the cancer had increased. Most troubling was that I didn't know why. When this tiny flea bit me, I feared for my life.

To help a friend escape the Florida heat, I had invited her to stay for a week with me that summer. She had brought her dog, Sugar, with her. Six days after they left, while I was sitting where Sugar slept, my ankle was bitten.

I went online praying that chemical bombs weren't as bad as I thought, but I discovered they were even worse. After I got radiation damage, and my body rejected the two medications, and I had the two lumpectomies that I now know weren't necessary, I promised myself I would never submit my body to harm again.

As ridiculous as this sounds even to myself, my first thought was that I either had to find a way to live with these little critters, or I had to use chemical bombs to get rid of them, which would make overcoming cancer take longer, cost me more, or perhaps become impossible.

"She died after getting fleas," I imagined my obituary reading, and I smiled. This brought me some much-needed relief, which allowed me to think more clearly. I had already taught myself that once I recognized a problem, it was my responsibility to solve it, not to indulge in fear or self-pity.

I Googled "natural ways to kill fleas" and found several websites with suggestions. All recommended vacuuming often, so I began vacuuming like crazy, sat down and rested, then vacuumed even more.

After my friend and her dog left, the weather had been hot and muggy, perfect weather for flea eggs to hatch. Blood is the only thing fleas eat and every female flea lays several hundred eggs after biting her host. Every time an egg hatched, these hungry fleas hunted me down.

My body was covered with flea bites. Even after vacuuming, I kept getting bitten, because once a flea is in your home, this is not your biggest problem: 50 percent is the eggs, 35 percent is the larvae, ten percent is the pupae, and only five percent is the fleas.

I got a migraine from all this stress and had to go to bed. I couldn't vacuum for 12 hours. My home became infested again, worse than before.

I questioned if what I was attempting was possible, so I asked my friends on Facebook for their suggestions. Here I learned that the only thing that kills fleas in all four stages of their lives is 100 percent orange essential oil. After purchasing as many cans as I could find, I sprayed the contents everywhere. I even slept armed with a bottle close to me at night because I kept being awakened by biting fleas. Six exhausting days later, after much vacuuming and spraying, my home was at last flea-free.

After several friends told me they would be furious if anyone's dog brought fleas into their home and they found it odd that I wasn't angry, I wondered why I wasn't. Maybe because for years I hated having a temper, so now I refused to get angry at all, even if it was appropriate. Or perhaps it was because I thought of myself as damaged goods and I had to be extra good just to be on a level playing field. Or maybe because ten years ago, my friend Bill had invited me to Bosnia with a group he was organizing for a friend to see "Our Lady of Medjugorje," and this redefined love for me.

A generous woman had paid to take 16 people on this pilgrimage so we would experience the love she felt every year she went. When I returned home, my heart had expanded so much from the love I felt, it hurt for days. From this, I recognized my heart had the capacity to feel and hold more love. Since I could feel my body contract every time I felt anger and this restricted love from flowing, I refused to be angry for a long time.

Once I understood that my heart could feel and hold more love, something in me changed: I saw my past differently. I realized how ridiculous I had been trying to get Gary, my mother, and my siblings to open their hearts. I saw that my job wasn't to interfere with whatever path they or anyone else chose to follow. Who was I to say they weren't exactly where they were supposed to be? I focused on accepting them and everyone as they were, just as I deserved and wanted to be accepted by all people.

I must take this one step further before I explain how this ties into my getting fleas. It's only natural for people to have conflicts. What defines our lives and our relationships is how we resolve them. When I'm hurt and confused by someone's behavior, I'll often ask them to help me understand them. Some people are happy to explain themselves and thank me because I cared enough to give them this opportunity to clarify themselves. Other people have become defensive and have turned the tables on me, accusing me of hurting them just because I wanted to understand them better and protect our relationship.

People are individuals and act accordingly: Two friends told me I was a dear friend for not getting angry. If their home had become infested with fleas, they said they would never allow this irresponsible person into their home again, which was something I never once considered.

After giving this much thought, I decided the most loving thing I could do for both Sugar's owner and me was to tell her that she was welcome to visit anytime, but she could not bring her dog again. However, the possibility of her dog having fleas was something she refused to consider or even discuss. She acted insulted that I would suggest such a thing.

I knew I had come from a fair and loving place, and I heard how this was received. My friend showed no interest in my perspective. The only thing she cared about was what she believed. How do people think it's possible to have a healthy relationship with anyone if they show no desire *to relate?*

I had long ago decided I could no longer afford to be treated like this. And I could no longer make these sacrifices for others. For the sake of my health and happiness, I could no longer tolerate people who showed no respect or interest in what I believed. And just like Lori had long ago told me, I had to stop this costly habit of seeing people as kinder than they showed themselves to be.

To strengthen my immune system, I had been avoiding everything that would compromise it for years, but I had been allowing people's self-serving behavior to compromise my health and happiness. No more.

Thank God that those irritating little beasts invaded my home, because they got me to see that my allegiance and loyalty had been misplaced once again. When we mold ourselves into being what others want us to be, we make it far more difficult to be happy and to heal ourselves. Since my goal was to forever improve my health, I had to treat myself with love and respect, especially when others didn't.

Turning Things to Your Advantage

Five neurologists told me I would die, and I turned this to my advantage. I knew that all five had been wrong, and I used this to support my decision to choose a natural treatment and decline the mastectomy. I also turned having fleas into a path for acquiring significant information. And, after my life felt threatened because my neurologist was thinking too myopically, and what the hospital offered was too restricted, I found a way to use my dissatisfaction with the medical care I was receiving to my advantage.

Write down negative experiences in your past and present that you turned around and used to your advantage.

_____

_____

_____

_____

_____

_____

_____

Write down negative experiences where you got stuck in this bleakness. What did this cost you and what might you do differently in the future?

_____

_____

_____

_____

_____

_____

_____

22

Trauma Symptoms Don't Just Go Away

Though at the time I had no idea what symptoms from trauma looked like, after I was diagnosed with radiation damage, I now realize I'd begun showing symptoms in the mid-90s. I had been terrified that my brain had been damaged by my treatment; that this was man-made. I was scared because the radiation damage wasn't something I was born with. Like the brain tumor, I hadn't lived with it all my life.

From this stress, I developed digestive issues. It was years before I could eat comfortably. My jaw used to clench so tightly at night that I lost two teeth and damaged more, which required thousands of dollars of dental work that I couldn't afford to have.

Because our bodies remember our past, my body was always prepared to run from any perceived danger. Even today, I have to remind myself to uncurl my toes because they dig into the surface below me, ready to help me flee if needed.

Until I was aware that I had become hyper-vigilant, my defensiveness had grown to feel normal to me. If anyone were to suggest differently, I was quick to lash out in defense (ironically proving their point). For years, there was no place I could go where I felt safe, because wherever I went, the memories I held within my body always came along with me.

I now do yoga three times a week, which helps me to relax. I meditate every morning and frequently meditate throughout the day, which helps to regulate my nervous system. I'm out the door by 7:00 a.m. to enjoy a long and invigorating walk.

We were all born longing to be seen, understood, loved, nurtured, and protected, but traumas leave us confused and unsure of ourselves.

The most destructive thing that traumas do is to disconnect us from ourselves and from others. Until I understood this, I didn't know why I preferred being alone, even though I was lonely. I felt separated from the world, living on the outside, watching as others enjoyed their lives. I spent decades isolated in my home because traumas left me feeling like there was nowhere I could go where I could fit in.

I had lost my ability to feel comfortable in my skin and in the presence of others, while at the same time I craved being able to connect with others. This is another reason it's vital to our healing that we have family and friends who understand this and will comfort and support us. We need people to tell us the reason we act so frightened is because our traumas blind us. We don't have the ability to understand this on our own. Many people, like me, spend years retreating in fear, experiencing loneliness and sadness.

If people who have been traumatized are belittled and judged harshly, additional damage will occur, and the longer their traumas will affect them.

Typical of someone who's been traumatized, I used to shame myself for not healing faster. I lived in fear that people would get upset and turn on me because the effects of the traumas lingered so long. Unintentionally, I delayed my healing by shaming myself and retreating into the safety of my home.

Until I understood the effects of all the traumas I had experienced, I had no idea my defensive behavior was typical of someone who had been traumatized. I didn't know that help was available to me, so I just kept adapting the best I could.

Christiane Northrup, OB/GYN physician and author of the book, *Women's Bodies, Women's Wisdom*, said it was natural for someone who has had a health scare to be emotionally affected for a long time after.

I thought I should have been able to overcome any problem I had. I shamed myself for years until I learned that our bodies need time after experiencing "the shocks and bumps and bruises" as Dr. Northrup called the traumas we experience. We need time to process all we've been through before our bodies fully heal.

What made my healing more challenging was that I kept experiencing additional "shocks, and bumps and bruises" as the symptoms from the radiation damage kept surfacing. And, as they did, my family's anger escalated. This not only created more problems for me, but it kept this cycle of trauma going.

After what I'd been through, I denied being traumatized because I needed to minimize what happened to me, for both my sake and my family's. This tactic protected me from getting overwhelmed. And I thought if I downplayed this, my family would feel more comfortable and perhaps they would accept me again. It wasn't until a friend asked me to define trauma for her did I have to admit that I'd been traumatized quite a few times. Once I accepted this, the healing from these traumas could at last begin.

Soldiers who have seen battle have shown that until they receive professional help and support from their families, their lives can and usually do fall apart. And yet trauma in our homes and hospitals is really no different. If we play down their significance and shame ourselves when symptoms appear, they will continue to harm us. Please learn from my mistake.

As studies of the mind/body connection have shown, our emotions affect our bodies in physical ways: when we imagine biting into a lemon, our mouths salivate, and when we see a policeman in our car's rearview mirror, our hearts may beat rapidly. A serious illness affects our bodies far more than biting into a lemon or seeing a policeman can, and our bodies respond accordingly. Believing or pretending our problems are behind us only embeds these problems deeper into our bodies, where they can do more damage to our lives.

For years, I told myself I should just be grateful that I was alive. While there are many benefits to being appreciative, I used being grateful to hide from my pain, not knowing that this would cause me more. It's natural for people to never want to revisit a painful experience. People often avoid having to think about it, but this also comes at a high cost.

I didn't understand that my hypervigilance and defensiveness were my body's way of telling me that I needed help. In hindsight, I couldn't face anything else being wrong with me or that maybe I really "wasn't right in my head," as my mother used to often yell at me.

Dr. Northrup also cited studies that showed when people were in remission from cancer, this was when they often lost their ability to enjoy life. To fully free ourselves from trauma, our fears must be faced, but this can only happen when we're ready and able.

As difficult as it was to hear that I had a brain tumor and would soon die, that I had radiation damage and could die in seconds, that I had breast cancer or that I had to get a mastectomy, my biggest challenges always came after.

Much of my life has been like a game of Whac-a-Mole. One problem wouldn't yet be resolved before another occurred, causing additional trauma. I wished I had reached out and gotten help sooner, but until I was aware that I needed help and help was available, I simply couldn't.

As the baby in my family, I was continually told to grow up and stop whining. This probably contributed to why, after five doctors told me I would die, not one doctor or anyone saw me cry. Another reason I went into the "I've got to be strong" mode was because there were no emotionally stable adults for me to rely on when I was growing up. I had to learn to be responsible. And once I overcame the breast cancer, I was more than ready to believe all my health problems were behind me. Admitting to myself that I had more work to do was beyond my capabilities.

When I lived with Gary, knowing his drugs took priority over my comfort and happiness made me realize I couldn't rely on him either. I stuffed my fears away and told myself I had to be strong. As my health problems continued, my fears naturally escalated, because this is what unresolved emotions do until they scream for our attention. The more I had to be strong, the less attention I could give my fears, and as time passed, the louder they screamed to be acknowledged.

In 2015, I heard Dr. Northrup say, "We are beginning to teach people to love and accept themselves and be with our bodies. And that it's okay to feel whatever we feel. We completely underestimate how powerful this is." As difficult as this is at times, remember that our discomfort and fears are meant to be felt.

Even though Lori taught me how important it was to feel my feelings, until I was ready and capable of feeling the depth of this pain, I couldn't. And as my pain and fears grew, this became more challenging.

Dr. Stephen Porges' Polyvagal Theory has been credited with having done more to improve our ability to heal, grow, and thrive than anything else in the past 50 years. From studying his work, I understood that my body had been reacting as it should in response to my past. From him I learned, "There is no such thing as a 'bad' response. There are only adaptive responses." Since Gary and my family were incapable of emotionally supporting me, I had been adapting the best way I could since I was first diagnosed in 1986.

With time, I taught myself to embrace myself with love and compassion *however* I acted, and to accept there was a reason I acted as I did. Once I began giving myself the love and support I needed, it took time and determination to break my habit of shaming and criticizing myself, but I succeeded.

"Safety turns off the defenses of our autonomic nervous system. Safety is the treatment," Dr. Porges said, which is why we need to surround ourselves with people who create a safe and loving environment for us, and to also give this to ourselves.

Once I stopped judging myself, and treated myself with love and compassion instead, regardless of how I acted, I created the safe and loving environment I had been craving for years. And from this state, I was able to grieve my losses—particularly the person I once was and the dreams that I had.

Before I got the brain tumor, I had no doubt I would get married, have children, and create a successful art career. I was sure I would never have to spend a holiday alone. But once I felt safe again another significant change occurred: I fully embraced my "after brain tumor life." Now I could celebrate who I was and my present life.

We all live in a grief-avoiding culture, which makes it more challenging for us to grieve. I had been carrying more grief than I realized, which made healing even more difficult. I had no idea that grief could have so many layers; that what I previously felt had only been the very top.

I had gone to great lengths to be a positive person, believing this was the healthiest thing to do before I recognized it was more important to be authentic with my feelings. I had been pulling a U-Haul behind me that was overflowing with grief and weighing me down. I had to stop and feel my pain and allow myself to grieve.

If I had received the support that my body needed, I don't think I would have lived so long in a protective mode. No doubt, if I was relaxed, my body would have been in a stronger position to fight the radiation damage. Or maybe I wouldn't have gotten the radiation damage at all, or perhaps my body would not have been damaged to the extent it was. Who knows?

If, after my doctor told me I had a life-threatening brain tumor, Gary had been able to consider my fear rather than make demands on me to satisfy his own needs, I have no doubt I would have felt safer. When I called my father to ask about his mother who died of a brain tumor, I wish he'd had the ability to consider the pain and trauma he caused by hanging up on me.

If my mother had been capable of comforting me in the hospital when I learned my life was threatened for a second time, or if my sister could have first thought about how scared I was from having breast cancer—*before* she hung up the phone—I'm sure my body would never have become so traumatized. If my brother had been capable of simply discussing with me that I had a brain tumor or radiation damage or breast cancer, instead of yelling out of a need to protect himself, I am sure my healing would have benefited. If any of my loved ones had been capable of giving me emotional support by offering their love rather than reacting out of fear, there is no question in my mind that this would have made a significant difference to my life.

If I hadn't felt so guilty about upsetting everyone by becoming sick, if I had not acquiesced to my mother's wishes, and if I had stopped shaming myself and being critical of myself much earlier, this would have assisted my healing as well.

It took me a long time to accept that how my loved ones were acting was not because of anything I did; that I was not to blame for their actions. It was years before I realized I didn't have the ability to make anyone act in any way, as silly as this now sounds to me. It was a while before I could grasp that the members of my family didn't have the ability to act any differently than they did, in much the same way I couldn't face the deeper levels of my grief until I could. Years passed before I understood that because my loved ones never learned how to regulate their nervous systems to help calm themselves, my getting sick was probably like me yelling "fire" while they felt trapped in a burning building.

When our emotions overwhelm us, like a drowning swimmer can only focus on saving himself, we can only consider our own needs. We can't think beyond ourselves because our ability to think becomes grossly restricted. Even after I understood this intellectually, it took longer emotionally. It took me years to realize that Gary and the members of my family weren't intentionally being cruel to me.

None of my loved ones were uncaring people: Gary had come to the clinic out of concern for me, and my mother had gone to the hospital to give me support. My sister agreed to be available after my doctor called me. The problem was that none of them were emotionally *able* to support me, and adding to this problem was that they all thought they could.

Imagine if Gary had never come to the clinic and I didn't have to cope with the additional problems he created. Imagine if my mother hadn't insisted on coming to the hospital and Gainor had come instead, or if my sister had suggested I call a friend who could support me instead of agreeing to be there for me. Imagine if Gary or any of the members of my family had been able to say, "We're going to beat this together." Or if any of them had been capable of simply asking, "What can I do for you?"

How different my life would have been, but their lack of self-awareness made this impossible. They all believed they could be supportive, and because they couldn't be, they did more harm than good. And then they got angry at me for exposing their deficiencies and causing them discomfort. People have often asked me if I have forgiven Gary and my family. I used to say it took me a while, but I have. However, today I think there's nothing to forgive because they were simply acting like themselves, doing the best they could with the tools they had. Just like me, they too had been influenced by their past and their bodies remembered this. Because they had not yet realized how much their past had harmed and influenced them, they made no effort to heal. This has caused them far more problems than it ever has or could for me.

***

In a *Law and Order* episode, Olivia stopped the young college student, Sarah, from running out of a courtroom after her rapist was found not guilty. Sarah was livid that she had gone through the trial for nothing. Because Olivia was emotionally grounded, she had the ability to connect, support, and comfort the highly agitated Sarah.

She told Sarah that punishing him wasn't going to help. That healing began when someone bore witness. Olivia looked at Sarah in the eyes and said that she saw and believed in her.

When I heard this, the hairs on my arms stood up, and I got chills. My eyes watered before I intellectually understood why my body was responding this way. When I heard that Olivia did not take Sarah's anger personally, but comforted her in a loving and compassionate way, my body reacted to what I had yearned to hear for almost 30 years: I had wanted to be seen, believed and understood. Finally, my body felt safe enough to feel the years of embedded pain I had been holding inside me and to release it.

"I saw you. I believe you," Olivia said to Sarah.

Simply hearing this after years of feeling unheard and unseen by my family allowed my body to heal, too.

Why We Need Support

For over a decade, I showed signs of trauma without realizing I was living in a protective survival mode. I was disconnected from myself and oblivious that I was. Once we are traumatized, we need others' help. Unfortunately, traumas also disconnect us from others. We no longer feel comfortable among people. Often, we fail to seek the help we need. If you have or have had a life-threatening disease, you have been traumatized. Please get help for yourself.

Google "signs of trauma" and make a list of these symptoms. Print the list out and learn each symptom. Identify and address each time that you show one.

Write down each time a trauma symptom surfaced. Did you get triggered and why? What did you tell yourself? How might you have handled the situation better?

_____

_____

_____

_____

_____

_____

_____

_____

_____

_____

_____

_____

_____

_____

_____

_____

23

Widening Your Perspective is a Must

"What does thinking outside the square mean?" I asked a friend, who chuckled at how I had "re-created" a common expression.

"You just did it, Sandi. You can't help yourself. You just naturally think outside the box," he said.

I was a teenager when I first understood the advantage of expanding the way I thought. I recognized the importance of understanding a wide variety of people's perspectives. I knew my relationships would improve if people felt heard and respected.

I realized that my perspective was limited. If I only saw things from my viewpoint, this would impede my growth and my thinking would remain shallow and underdeveloped.

"In the end, it cannot be doubted that each of us can only see part of the picture," Dr. Paul Kalanithi wrote in his insightful book, *When Breath Becomes Air*, while he was dying from lung cancer.

"The doctor sees one, the patient another, the engineer a third, the economist a fourth, the pearl diver a fifth, the alcoholic a sixth, the cable guy a seventh, the sheep farmer an eighth, the Indian beggar a ninth, the pastor a tenth. Human knowledge is never contained in just one person. It grows from the relationships we create between each other and the world, and it never is complete."

I was in my boyfriend's college dormitory when I first read the following quote from Socrates: "The only true wisdom is in knowing you know nothing." Typical of a curious young adult, I thought about this often and from many angles.

What particularly frightened me after doctors diagnosed me with the brain tumor was that people I thought I needed, despite being extremely intelligent—such as my neurologist and Gary—had not yet learned to think in this deeper, more inclusive way.

Paul Cézanne, one of the most influential artists of the twentieth century, showed how much he understood this through his art. He knew that none of us could truly see something from our one and thereby limited perspective. To give himself and his viewers a clearer understanding of what he painted, he would shift from one foot to the other and sway back and forth.

In 1977, I received a full scholarship from the Leo Marchutz School of Painting and Drawing in Aix-en-Provence, France. Here I was given this opportunity to study where Cézanne was born and painted many of his magnificent masterpieces. In the same spots where he once worked, I joyfully painted from the same motifs. When I returned home, I incorporated Cezanne's multidimensional way of understanding into my life by putting extra effort into learning and respecting how others thought.

And yet it's quite humbling when I think of how long it took me to distinguish between what I'm responsible for and what I'm not; to know that what other people say and how they act is their responsibility and not mine.

Until I was in my early 40s, if someone got angry with me, I felt mortified, responsible, and embarrassed. Believing I must have done something wrong, I would apologize immediately. And yet every time I got angry, I felt responsible and guilty. I spent years believing I was guilty both ways and shamed myself unmercifully.

Taking responsibility for myself and others added to my exhaustion after I got sick. It wreaked havoc on my body and health. And I felt horrible for all the pain I caused my loved ones by getting a brain tumor and a temper. When I got radiation damage, I lived with nagging guilt because I thought I was responsible for my family becoming furious. Once I understood that my responsibility was only for what I said and how I acted, this huge pressure was lifted.

Viktor Frankl wrote, "Between stimulus and response, there is a space. In that space lies our power to choose our response. In our response lies our growth and freedom."

By stopping myself from habitually reacting to others' anger, and no longer blaming myself for it, I created for myself this space that Frankl wrote about. By becoming a witness, I taught myself to decipher what I was and wasn't accountable for.

This was also how I stopped myself from having the temper the brain tumor had given me. And for the first time, I could consciously understand that Gary, my mother, and my brother also had tempers, but none of them ever took responsibility for theirs. Because I had been feeling so guilty, I never thought about this before: None of them seemed to care that they lost control and yelled at me, and they didn't have a brain tumor as an excuse. They never apologized to me, as I always did every time I lost control and yelled back at each of them.

"Everything changes once we identify with being the witness to the story, instead of the actor in it," wrote Ram Dass, American spiritual teacher, psychologist, and author.

By stepping back and creating this space, I gave myself the ability to view life through a wider lens and see the bigger picture.

While a prisoner in Auschwitz, Frankl observed that the human spirit was "mighty powerful." And thoughts were the one thing the Germans could not take from any inmate. He noticed that those who found things to appreciate throughout their days were not only the happiest and the healthiest, but they even lived the longest.

"Everything can be taken from a man but one thing: the last of human freedoms—to choose one's attitude in any given set of circumstances, to choose one's own way," Frankl wrote.

After I read this, during my most challenging times, I told myself if prisoners in a concentration camp could be this disciplined under their inhumane circumstances, I could be too.

Five years before I read Frankl's book, I dedicated three months to painting the mural to express the importance of appreciating life. Despite receiving hundreds of letters of thanks, three people wrote to tell me they knew what my personal view on life should be and what I ought to be expressing and sharing through my art.

This piqued my curiosity. What makes certain people think others should think like they do, and why do some people need to criticize those who think differently, especially an artist expressing herself? What made it impossible for a person to not recognize that we are all individuals, that we all have different experiences, and we will naturally not all think alike? Why can some people think and understand this multi-dimensional way of thinking from a young age while some adults never do?

"Death is the type of thing that, it seems like people aren't able to express in a worldly sense, so the mural was very thought-provoking to me. This has the depth that could be discussed in a philosophy class for months. You have made a great impact on many people," a high school student wrote to me.

Every religion recommends that we open and extend ourselves to others, and that this enriches our lives. So, what is it that stops some people from recognizing this and respecting how others think?

In Frankl's words, "in our response lies our growth and our freedom."

Numerous studies have shown that the emotional development of children who grow up around addictions and in dysfunctional families is stunted. Until we stop and recognize this correlation, adult children will continue to act the same way they were taught by adults in their home who struggled emotionally.

Prisoners in concentration camps would have been justified if they had felt anger and bitter for being forced to live in their inhumane circumstances, but there were some who chose not to live this way. Whether you have a life-threatening brain tumor, cancer, or any other challenge, or even if you are perfectly healthy, how you respond to life influences your health and happiness.

I had been having trouble accepting people who thought they knew all there was to know and yet I believe that everyone has a right to think however they choose. I laughed at myself when I realized that I was restricting myself with my own narrow thinking.

Choosing How You Want to Live

My family was imprisoned by their feelings. Similarly, the way I responded to my family weakened me until I decided "no more." I decided if prisoners in a concentration camp could be disciplined, I could too. I taught myself to regulate my nervous system. And you can as well.

Learn to regulate your nervous system. Use the tools in this book or find help elsewhere.

Write down each time you failed to regulate your nervous system and you got triggered. Write down what challenged you, and why you came unglued. What did this cost you? And how might you respond better in the future?

_____

_____

_____

_____

_____

_____

_____

_____

_____

_____

_____

_____

_____

_____

_____

_____

_____

24

Be Grateful for Even Small Things Everyday

Thanks to the discovery of the Magnetic Resonance Imaging Machine (MRI), there is now evidence that shows that when gratitude is practiced, new pathways form in our brains. Using gratitude, I formed new pathways in my brain which assisted and enhanced my life.

I used to get frustrated by all the setbacks I kept having, feeling like Sisyphus, who was forced for eternity to roll a boulder up a hill, only to have it roll back down again. Gratitude saved and strengthened me because every time I felt grateful, I felt love.

Feeling appreciative wasn't always possible. Every time I had a migraine, I certainly didn't feel grateful. However, having these migraines proved we don't have to feel grateful 100 percent of the time to reap the many benefits of gratitude. Sometimes screaming in frustration is the healthiest thing to do, since we all need to vent at times.

A car is a great place to do this. Feeling frustrated one hot summer day while driving to my studio, I screamed in my car as loud as I could. This was during a time I couldn't afford to own a car with air conditioning, and I had forgotten that my windows were rolled down.

On the sidewalk stood a small-framed elderly man, stooped over his cane, who had stopped for a moment to rest. When he heard me scream, his head jerked up and his two eyes bulged as he frantically searched to see who was being murdered. Lesson learned: be sure your car windows are rolled up *before* you scream in frustration.

***

Melody Beattie, author of self-help books on codependent relationships, wrote, "Gratitude unlocks the fullness of life. It turns what we have into enough, and more. It turns denial into acceptance, chaos to order, confusion to clarity. It can turn a meal into a feast, a house into a home, a stranger into a friend. Gratitude makes sense of our past, brings peace for today, and creates a vision for tomorrow."

Anne Kubitsky, who is a speaker, activist, and the founder of the school program, "Look for the Good Project," teaches the importance of being grateful. She has proven that gratitude impacts school children and the climate in which they learn. Once gratitude is incorporated into their lives, children's ability to learn and their self-esteem increases, while their stress levels decrease.

Feeling appreciative helped me heal my broken heart and my damaged body, much like a jumper cable brings life back to a dead car battery. It heightened my senses by saturating me with bursts of uplifting energy that boosted me.

I used to lie in bed and list things that I appreciated in alphabetical order. If I got to the letter "Z" and I didn't feel more relaxed, I would go through the alphabet a second time, listing more things I appreciated. This helped me make the most of what I had, despite my ongoing problems. Gratitude helped me accomplish all I did. By appreciating, accepting, and allowing life to happen without insisting things go my way, stuck wheels got greased, making life much easier.

**

"To thine own self be true," William Shakespeare wrote.

I read that Louise Hay, internationally renowned author of *You can Heal Your Life*, believed that breast cancer represents putting everyone else first, which had always been my problem, due to my lack of self-worth and my desire to be loved. Because my mother suffered from trigeminal neuralgia, I told her that Louise Hay believed that since our face is what we show the world and if problems occur here, we need to find ways to feel safe and truthfully express who we are. My mother laughed and told me I was being absurd. But when we are true to ourselves and express our needs, that's how we help our healing, as I discovered from my own experience. But my mother's beliefs differed from mine, and I had to accept this.

When I moved back to New England from Washington D.C. in 1989, I brought my dearly loved cat, Buster, with me. When I first found him, a sick and helpless stray, he gratefully followed me everywhere.

"That cat is in love with you," my mother said when she saw us together. She began getting up earlier in the morning before I awoke so she could feed Buster, but when this didn't successfully steal his love from me, she said, "I thought cats always preferred the person who feeds them. Buster's loyalty is only to you, probably because you act like you're the Queen of England."

My mother viewed me like this because I had learned to take care of myself. She had never learned to be true to herself or appreciate the woman she was, so she resented me when I began to take good care of myself to help my body heal. After I got sick, I focused on what my body needed, and my mother never stopped fighting me about this. She even called me selfish and railed against how I was using love as my guide and following my intuition because I would not do as she demanded.

Every human being has been created with their own internal GPS—an intuition—but our intuition doesn't always feel consistent. Sometimes my intuition feels subtle, and I have to stop and concentrate to get a good read on it. Living in our heads and ignoring our bodies makes this even more challenging, though most people can feel when something isn't right. They become uncomfortable and may not be able to identify why, but they do know when something feels off.

There are other times when my intuition speaks so loudly that there is no way I can overlook what it's telling me. At other times, my intuition may feel tranquil, more like a nurturing and loving feeling, as if everything is right in the world. Other times, I have become so passionate about something that I have no doubt about what I need to do, such as using a natural treatment to heal when I had breast cancer, painting the mural, and writing this book.

What I found interesting—and comforting—was that the angrier my family got with me, the louder my inner voice spoke, protecting me in such a loving and caring manner. In this way, my family helped me grow more confident in trusting my ability to feel and believe what my intuition was telling me. And it confirmed that my body was protecting me, even from my family's anger. Listening and having faith in my intuition was imperative to saving my life.

My body proved it remembers the past, even experiences that were minor: I was painting in my studio one day listening to Michael McDonald singing "Ain't No Mountain High Enough." The next day, I placed my paintbrush in the same spot on my canvas where I had stopped painting the day before and Michael McDonald's voice began singing the same song again.

I looked up to see who had turned on my music, but no one was there. When I realized that the music was coming from inside me, I wondered if I carried this music inside my body, and what else was I unknowingly carrying that might be weighing me down? And could this additional weight be contributing to the migraines?

Despite my health improving, the migraines continued for almost three decades, leaving me exhausted to such a degree that I could no longer wear boots in the winter, or the heavy malachite necklace from Africa my brother had given me before I got sick, because they wore me out. Vacuuming was practically impossible. It had to be done in short spurts, which was also how I managed to wash my dishes.

"Our brains use 25 percent of our body's energy. Yours, to heal itself, is using more. Your brain is using more energy and, on top of this, you're getting migraines too. I'm surprised you're able to do all you do," one doctor told me, but could offer me no help.

The Imitrex I took did stop the pain, but the migraines still pummeled my body. I had been doing all I could to discourage them, but nothing worked. After I questioned what other things might be weighing me down, to encourage energy to flow more freely by opening up clogged constrictions, I tried Reiki, acupuncture, meditation, massage, chiropractic care, writing, yoga, art—any technique someone offered me for free or at a discount—and each one inched me forward.

Not many years ago, I was at a party and got a terrible migraine. I told my friend Jessica I had to leave before I threw up. Once outside, she suggested I come to her house and wrap myself in her Solaris blanket.

"It reflects your body's energy back onto you," she explained.

All I wanted to do was to get home and climb into bed. She gave me a key to her home and invited me to wrap myself in her blanket anytime. Despite having doubts, the next time I felt a migraine starting while I was driving near her home, I did as she suggested. To my surprise, the migraine stopped within 20 minutes. After this worked a second time, I bought my own blanket and I now sleep with it every night. I've never had a migraine again. (You can read more about this on my website www.sandigold.com.)

Scott Kiloby, author, speaker, and expert on mindfulness, and co-founder of the Kiloby Inquiries, believes, "At some point in our lives, most of us unconsciously developed contractions, which are like blocked energies occurring in the head, throat, chest and heart area, stomach, pelvic or root area."

Scott believes we develop contractions, "when we are faced with perceived psychological threats, rejection, or trauma from childhood, albeit in a more unconscious way. Even if the body doesn't visibly contract, the contractions are formed. For some of us, addictions develop as a way to further cope with this buried pain. By medicating these areas, we get to continue to not have to feel these buried emotions. But addictions are only temporary fixes. They cover up the pain. They don't deal with the underlying issues."

I developed a sharp pain in my right shoulder. After a physical therapist questioned and examined me, he explained that my problem occurred because I had been twisting my body as a protective reaction to repeated traumas. While lying on my back on his examining table, he scooted one arm and his upper body underneath my shoulder and upper back. He held me as my body slowly untwisted in a slow, jerking fashion.

"What are you doing?" I asked, alarmed by this strange movement.

"I'm not doing anything. Your body's intelligence is. Your body is responding to the support I'm giving it. Our bodies love us, Sandi. They're always trying to help us, but only when they feel safe can we most efficiently heal."

Anthropologist Helen Fisher believes our brains are wired to love and be loved. I believe this includes developing a loving relationship with not just others, but with ourselves. This includes developing a love and appreciation for our body's intelligence, too.

What Helps the Flow to Flow?

I saw an acupuncturist who explained that needles unclog "traffic jams" that occur along our bodies' meridians. After experiencing different modalities, I recognized that finding ways to unclog these blocked areas (to make energy flow in my body the way energy was meant to flow) would help me. This is why I don't stay angry for long. I don't like the feeling of being clogged by my anger. This is why I eat the food my body likes. This is why I exercise, as well as why I have a European Thermography and an OA test every year. And why, after my doctor suggested it, I now get a massage every month.

Make a list of the ways you might help your energy to flow more freely in your body and your life.

_____

_____

_____

_____

_____

_____

_____

Make a list of the ways your energy has gotten blocked and where in your body you can feel this. What cost do you pay by allowing these "traffic jams" to remain?

_____

_____

_____

_____

_____

_____

_____

25

Sometimes You May Not Realize
How Stress is Affecting You

My brother emailed me, "Stress has become just the latest popular thing but it's highly over-rated." I was surprised that such an intelligent person hadn't yet recognized the effect stress had on his own body. I wondered if perhaps the harm stress does hadn't become as well-known to the public as I thought. I Googled "effect of stress" and found many articles. One was titled, "Chronic Stress Puts Your Health at Risk," published by the Mayo Clinic. It explained how chronic stress wreaks havoc on our bodies and our minds. When we are startled by a perceived threat, a small region in our brain (called the hypothalamus) sets off an internal alarm system, and this prompts our adrenal glands to release adrenaline and cortisol.

Was it possible my brother couldn't feel the effects from the cortisol as it surged through his body? Had he simply gotten used to this as a result of growing up with our melodramatic mother? Did he ever think about regulating his nervous system to help calm himself? Or did he perhaps like the feeling of this rush because of the power it gave him, since he hadn't learned a healthier way to empower himself?

It's fairly common knowledge that adrenaline increases our heart rate and elevates our blood pressure, and that cortisol is a stress hormone and increases glucose into the bloodstream, isn't it? But most people probably don't know that this can alter and suppress our immune system's response, which can compromise our digestive system, reproductive system, growth and healing.

My brother had digestive issues, and yet wouldn't a doctor have suggested that he improve the way he managed his stress?

When we experience long-term stress and we're exposed to stress hormones like cortisol and adrenaline for a long period of time, our risk of anxiety is increased, along with depression, heart disease, digestive problems, sleep problems, memory, and concentration. I wondered if my brother knew this.

Did he know that cortisol creates inflammation in our bodies, and that diseases like cancer thrive in this environment? My brother probably knew stress caused health problems but he had told himself that stress was overrated to avoid taking responsibility for his health.

Carl Jung said, "There is no coming to consciousness without pain. People will do anything, no matter how absurd, in order to avoid facing their own soul. One does not become enlightened by imagining figures of light, but by making the darkness conscious."

People who have become hypervigilant are at greater risk of long-term stressors, which cause them additional harm. So why didn't my oncologist tell me that stress could contribute to the breast cancer I had and that it was important I find ways to manage it?

This is yet another reason we must all advocate for ourselves and why a support system is crucial. I have found invaluable help online from Lynn Fraser, a meditator and a trauma survivor with more than 30 years' experience, who offers many free and effective ways to regulate our nervous systems and other insightful information that has helped me relax and improve my health and my life.

According to Google Scholar Citations, George P. Chrousos is on the list of 100 most cited scientists in the world. He is also among the 250 most prominent clinical investigators in the world. He wrote an article titled "Stress and Disorders of the Stress System" that defines stress as "a state in which homeostasis is actually threatened or perceived to be so."

I want to emphasize the words "perceived to be," meaning no one can tell someone what is and isn't stressful. If someone perceives something as a threat, it is threatening to them.

Once I understood that my family's inability to cope with my illness was because of a *perceived threat* that had ignited their nervous systems and distorted their thinking, this helped me to understand them better. Once I understood that their behavior was because of their need to protect themselves from fear, my stress levels decreased.

I used to live in fear of having the rug pulled out from beneath me because this happened so often in my past. Warning signs of danger used to scream in my head throughout each day from the many things I perceived as threatening, because not only had my health threatened me, but I felt threatened by people I had trusted my entire life. I even began to fear my friends at times who never meant any harm to me, which caused me to live in isolation for many years.

A 2015 article in *Science News* titled "Chronic stress can wreak havoc on the body: Finding a way to chill may benefit long-term health" stated: "Loneliness and other chronic stressors are particularly detrimental in people with cancer. The major cause of death from cancer is metastasis, when the disease spreads within our body. A test in mice with breast cancer showed that stress—induced by putting the animals in a confined space for two hours a day for 20 days—increased the likelihood of metastasis by 30-fold." Here is yet more proof about why love and support is needed—to help reduce our stress.

On a late Friday afternoon, at the end of a long and tiring week, I was looking forward to spending a quiet evening resting. I'd been using Bill Henderson's natural protocol to overcome breast cancer while working as an Expressive Arts Specialist for hospice. I loved my job, but the amount of driving to see each patient exhausted me. While ascending the stairs leading up to my condominium, I saw my neighbor, the president of our condominium association, looking down at me. I liked him. He was an older, tall, thin, kind, and gentle gray-haired man.

"I was just doing the yearly books," he said. "And it appears you've missed paying three months of condo fees."

"What?! There's got to be some mistake. You know I always pay on time. I'd rather go hungry than owe anyone money. Are you sure?"

"I check it off each month when I receive someone's monthly fee, but I could just as easily have made a mistake as you. Look in your checkbook and get back to me. No hurry."

I dashed into my condo and looked through my checkbook and scanned my bank statements. I was surprised to discover that this mistake was mine, after living here 134 months and always paying the condo fee on time. And yet, in less than one year, I'd forgotten to pay it three times.

"Don't worry about it, Sandi. I understand. We all make mistakes. I'm not closing the books for three months. Don't put extra pressure on yourself. There really is no need," he told me.

"That I can be this much out-of-touch is what I find most threatening. I thought I was handling having cancer well, but now I have to wonder what else I've forgotten. This is scary, especially because I live alone," I replied.

After a doctor tells his patients that they have cancer or any life-threatening disease, life naturally becomes more stressful for them. This upsets their body's chemical balance, which influences their thoughts and behavior. Regaining balance takes time and effort, especially if the threat is long-lasting. Please be patient with yourself.

When I made a mistake like this, I found it helpful to stop and ask myself how this had happened so I could make the appropriate change. Many people believe what triggered them caused their stress, but this keeps them from strengthening themselves so they're no longer being triggered by the same thing.

I also formed a habit of searching for the silver lining in every problem I had; when I forgot to pay my condo fees, I was pleased that I had reacted by being kind to myself instead of shaming myself for this mistake.

Life is stressful for most people. Many of us have several balls in the air that we're always juggling. Having a serious illness is also stressful because it requires even more from us. Living alone, getting migraines, and all the additional expenses from the radiation damage, followed by the costs from the breast cancer, were challenging. I had to learn not to make my life even more difficult.

I taught myself to have compassion for myself whenever I made a mistake. With each improvement that I made, I gave myself a positive reward, something to acknowledge I was improving. Following this conversation with my neighbor, despite being tired, I took a walk and enjoyed the support that nature gave me.

"Stress doesn't only make us feel awful emotionally," said Jay Winner, MD, author of *Take the Stress Out of Your Life*. "It can also exacerbate just about any health condition you can think of."

Getting cancer, or any illness, not only negatively impacts our bodies in physical ways, but it affects our moods, our sense of well-being, our confidence, and behavior. After I forgot to pay my condo fees, and after I got my brother's email and read about the many ways stress affects our bodies, I made it a conscious habit to better manage mine, since the mistake I had made proved I needed to do a better job.

By treating myself as if I was deserving of peace, by creating a safe and supportive environment for myself, and remembering to encourage myself like a loving mother would encourage her toddler whenever he made a mistake, my health and life continued to gradually improve.

As there was growing evidence showing how stress negatively affects the outcome of all diseases, it would have been far more advantageous if I had learned how to manage stress *before* I got sick—which I encourage all my readers to do. Wouldn't it be great if we were taught in elementary school how to regulate our nervous systems to help us all manage stress?

"I can't imagine what it's like being as sick as you've been, living alone and having to support yourself, especially as an artist. Call me anytime if ever you need me. I'm just minutes away," my friend Cathy told me. I felt both of my shoulders lower in response to the loving support my friend offered.

Don't Stress Over Stress

It's important to practice stress management. But whenever you are stressed, don't stress about this too. I used to worry about the amount of stress on my body, until I realized that this only contributed to the amount of stress I carried. I suggest meditating. If meditating isn't your thing, I'd find an online or in-person group before you rule it out. Meditating with others makes a big difference. Learning to regulate your nervous system is the key. However you learn to do this is up to you.

Make a list of the ways you can improve how you manage your stress.

_____

_____

_____

_____

_____

_____

_____

Keeping your focus on yourself, make a list of the times you got stressed and why. What might you have done or can do in the future to help decrease your stress? And, if you allow stress to hijack you, what cost are you paying?

_____

_____

_____

_____

_____

_____

_____

26

You Often Need to Nurture and Reassure Yourself

The most frightening thing every doctor said could happen never did. Continually being told all these gruesome possibilities, describing what my future might hold, had a negative effect on me. Outwardly, I appeared to be handling this well, but hearing all these grim prognoses did make me nervous. To help put an end to my anxiousness, I asked myself how many times would I keep responding in fear, when this had been proven to be unnecessary time and time again?

I noticed that every time I reacted in fear, and I resisted change, I suffered. To help myself break this habit, I first allowed myself to feel my fear and not shame myself for feeling it. Whenever I caught myself resisting anything at all, I practiced letting go by reminding myself I was alive and doing well *in this present moment.*

I told myself that even if I didn't get the comfort I deserved as a child or get the support I needed from my family after I got sick, I could give *myself* the loving reassurance that my body needed now. Empowering myself in this way made a significant difference.

I was given an opportunity to see how much I had grown and that I'd learned to take care of myself when I was working for hospice.

I got called into a meeting. One of the company's vice presidents was sitting across the table from a younger dark-haired woman who worked in human resources. No one else was there. I walked into the room feeling somewhat nervous, and the two women smiled.

"We want you to know we are very happy with the work you do and have heard only good things about you and that your patients love you.

However, I'm sorry to have to tell you that the company has made a mistake," the younger woman said.

The company made a mistake?

She continued, "We've been paying you as if you had your master's degree. Since you only have your bachelor's, we have to decrease your pay accordingly."

Surprised by the low figure she handed me on a slip of paper, I replied, "You are going to reduce my pay by almost half, despite my being a good employee, and having years of experience working for you?"

"We really are sorry."

"But I didn't lie on my resume. I was honest with you."

"We are taking full responsibility for this."

"Oh, you will? Then how about meeting me halfway and only reducing my pay by one quarter instead of half. This way, I won't be the only one being penalized. That's fair. Don't you think?"

"I'm sorry. We can't do that."

"Then how about if you pay for my schooling so I can get my master's?"

"But there is no Expressive Arts Specialist position available here for someone who has their master's."

"At least I'd have this degree, and you would have done something to make up for your mistake. No? Well, then let's talk about how long it will take to increase my pay from where you have now placed it, including my cost-of-living raises."

"We don't give raises to people who work in complementary care as you do."

"Never?"

"We never have, and we have no plans to."

"This is the first time I've been told this. So more bad news."

It was clear that I did not matter to this company. I had learned this from similar conversations with people who only wanted what they wanted. I knew I had to play the best cards that had been dealt to me. This didn't mean I liked it, or I thought it was fair—only that I'd learned when to stop beating my head against the wall. I sat with my chin lowered towards my chest, knowing that speaking would do me no good.

"I can't tell you how badly we feel. I can imagine what you must be feeling. We really wouldn't blame you if you want to get angry and vent," the woman from human resources said as she twirled a black pen in her hand.

"Getting angry would only create more stress for me, which wouldn't be healthy. I have breast cancer and I'm treating it using natural means.

Please don't think I'm saying this to guilt-trip you. That's not my style. I'm just explaining why I'm being quiet."

"You don't want to say anything?"

"I'm silently practicing stress management. I once had a brain tumor and the treatment gave me breast cancer. It helped me know that under all circumstances my responsibility is to take care of myself."

I could feel my body strengthen in response to my words. Encouraged by this, I continued, "I'm sitting here reminding myself that I've dealt with far more difficult things. Being sick has been quite costly. I would be a liar if I told you I'm not concerned about this reduction in pay, but what choice have you left me?"

"We really are so sorry."

"I love my job. I love my patients and I'm not about to walk out on them. I'm going to have to find ways to live on less ... You both look surprised. Do you want me to show you what I've learned that's helping me to cope?"

The younger woman glanced across the table at her superior, who nodded her consent. I asked if the younger woman would stand, and she rose from her chair. I could feel my body strengthen again as I took back control.

"First, I need to get a baseline, so we'll have something to compare. Extend one arm in front of you, at about shoulder height."

She did as I requested.

"In a moment, I'm going to ask you to close your eyes while I push your extended arm down. Notice how much resistance it takes to hold it up."

I gently pushed on her arm. It moved downward with some resistance. Then I instructed her to put both arms by her side and think negative thoughts with her eyes closed. Once this negativity saturated her body, I instructed her to extend her arm again, keeping her eyes shut, and notice her resistance when I pushed her arm this time.

Her arm quickly fell. She had no resistance. The woman's eyes opened wide in surprise. I then requested that she do the exact same thing, but think only positive thoughts this time. When I pushed on her extended arm, no matter how hard I pushed it, it was impossible for me to move it.

Both women stared at me in disbelief, as if I'd performed a magic trick.

"I've taught ways to help ourselves, including how our thoughts affect us, in hospitals, to people who have cancer and other illnesses, and in my art studio, to rape victims and people whose loved ones have died, because it's crucial for people to know that we all have this power."

Both women just stared and said nothing.

"Will you scream and shout when you get home?"

"Probably not. Maybe cry, though I doubt it. I don't want either of you to feel bad because that's not healthy either. I'm sure having to tell me this has been stressful for both of you."

Both women looked at me as though they didn't know what to say. A short period of silence followed until the younger woman apologized once again.

"Please don't feel bad and put more stress on yourself. That's the last thing I want. I like you and really don't want you to feel bad just because you have a job to do."

When she asked me how I taught myself to think like I do, I suggested four books: *The Four Agreements* by Don Miguel Ruiz, *Illusions* by Richard Bach, *Man's Search for Meaning* by Viktor Frankl, and *The Great Divorce* by C. S. Lewis.

The woman from HR dug into her brown leather purse to find a piece of paper and pen. She wrote these titles down while the older woman stared straight ahead with a frozen expression on her face. After both women thanked me for coming, I stood and walked out the door. Since it was the end of the workday, I went directly to the parking lot where, once inside my car, I laughed at my audaciousness.

"You've come a long way, baby!" I yelled, elated by how good it felt to break this lifelong habit of allowing others to define my happiness. I had finally freed myself, and my pride and confidence soared.

Once home, I called my old boss, who had left the company just two weeks before. She assured me that my salary had been equal to everyone else's in my position. Reducing people's salaries was the company's way of reducing costs.

Not long after, I also left, and was later told by a former co-worker that this same vice president had been abruptly fired. According to rumors, she'd been embezzling money from the company, though I have no way of knowing if this is true.

I know that she appeared to be an unhappy person, cold and aloof. Every hair on her head was perfectly in place and her makeup was so heavily applied it looked like a mask that seemed to say she couldn't accept who she was. Perhaps I was a victim of embezzlement, and she had taken my money, hoping it would buy her happiness. After I had gained as much as I had, how could I not feel sorry for her?

Reflect On and Celebrate Your Triumphs

Celebrating my victories was something I never even thought of doing until Lori suggested it. This is rewarding and fun. Some examples: you got your test results, and you are pleased. Celebrate! Someone screamed at you and you saw how distorted their face got. Because you didn't allow their anger to affect you, celebrate! How? Take yourself to the movies or buy yourself a piece of jewelry or whatever. Make growing and healing fun. Make a list of the fun ways you celebrated your triumphs. Know that you don't have to spend money. I often go for walks to reward myself or will relax while listening to music.

Write down each time you didn't reward yourself and why, and what this cost you. How does this feel and where in your body do you feel this?

_____

_____

_____

_____

_____

_____

_____

Write down each time you rewarded yourself and what this felt like and how this helped you.

_____

_____

_____

_____

_____

_____

_____

27

We Were All Created to Connect with Others

I have written a book that I would have found helpful when I was struggling and in need of answers. While I wrote it primarily to benefit people who have a life-threatening disease, it's really not just for people who have health problems. Since we all benefit when we treat ourselves lovingly and share our love with others, this book shows how love affects the outcome of our healing *and* our entire lives.

Every person responds in a favorable way to love—physically, emotionally, and spiritually. Our healing process accelerates when we feel loved and supported and when we open our hearts and share our love with others.

Despite the war on cancer and the billions of dollars the United States alone has spent to eliminate it, we haven't succeeded. If people took the necessary steps to discourage illness from occurring—by treating themselves and others in a loving manner—far fewer people would get sick. If those who did use their illnesses as reminders to love themselves and others, they would get healthier faster. And the world would be a happier place. By incorporating more love into all of our lives, not only would our lives improve, but the number of people who die from illnesses would also be reduced.

Years before I was diagnosed with a brain tumor, Dr. Bernie Siegel, a retired surgeon from the Yale-New Haven Hospital and best-selling author, humanized medical care by talking, listening, and learning from his patients. He has written extensively about patients who accelerated their healing process, using the healing power of love and positive thoughts. At first, he was laughed at and ridiculed by his peers.

Bernie has repeatedly stated that, "A vigorous immune system can overcome cancer if it is not interfered with. Emotional growth toward greater self-acceptance and fulfillment helps keep the immune system strong."

Dr. Bernie Siegel writes in his book *Love, Medicine and Miracles*, published in 1986, that love has proven to have a powerful effect on our immune system. He confirmed my belief in the healing power of love and influenced my decision to use love to guide me. If my doctors had read his book and learned from him, and if my family and Gary had been aware of their behavior and cared about how it affected me (and knew how it affected their own lives), my life would have turned out differently.

Dying didn't feel like "a fit" to me, though I certainly thought about it. I had told Gary that if I died he shouldn't feel guilty when he dated again because I wanted him to be happy and always to be loved.

Some friends insisted I was in denial when I was first diagnosed with the brain tumor, so I decided the responsible thing would be to consider their beliefs. I closed my eyes and visualized my friends and family gathering in remembrance of me on East Dock in Groton Long Point. But so many people were there, the dock collapsed and fell into the water. I interpreted this to mean that my body was telling me my funeral would not be happening anytime soon.

When someone is first diagnosed with a life-threatening disease, it's not unusual for her to shut down and go numb. Some people go into denial, though denial isn't necessarily a bad thing because it's the way our bodies protect us from becoming overwhelmed.

Some people, when first diagnosed with cancer, will panic. They may not be able to talk, think, eat, or sleep for days. Others may want to be left alone, while some will want to be surrounded by people. If a loved one appears to be in denial, they are probably in this protective state to shield themselves. Tearing this off before they are ready can in fact do them harm.

Having breast cancer was far less life-threatening than having a brain tumor, but I found it to be more frightening. I could have had my right breast cut off, but chopping off my head was never an option. When someone discovers she has cancer, there is no wrong way to act despite what others may believe. It's harsh and inappropriate to judge how people respond after they've been terrorized.

After learning that someone has cancer, when are they more deserving of love and support? Everyone benefits when we open our hearts and share our love and compassion with one another, so why would you not help others? Even if someone needs to scream and vent their rage at God, you, and everyone else, it's crucial that they be allowed to do this because it assists their immune systems and helps their body heal.

Unless you are someone who feels more secure when others take charge, and you don't believe in using your God-given intuition, then you may feel comfortable having someone else run your life. Since I know my body better than anyone can, I am someone who wants to be in charge. I view this as my right and my responsibility. I found being ill an enlightening, life-changing experience that affected me in many positive ways.

Because I kept my heart open, being sick made me a better, wiser, and happier person. If I had focused on my pain and losses, blamed others for how I felt, sat on the pity pot until I got a bright red ring, and done what everyone told me to do, I am sure I would not be alive today. I certainly wouldn't be the woman I have grown to be.

Because symptoms from the radiation damage continued to surface for decades I only had a small window of time to accomplish what I needed to do cach day. Every time I got a migraine, this allotted time decreased. Keeping myself as healthy as possible had to be my priority. After I got breast cancer, this required even more time and gave me an even smaller window to do what was needed. Because my time was limited and precious, I had to learn what was important and what wasn't. And whose company I could afford to keep.

Being as sick as I was and for such a long time helped me become the person I was created to be. If I had acquiesced to other people and acted how they wanted, if I hadn't followed my heart and chosen love as my guide, I wouldn't have been able to keep myself alive.

When Are You More Deserving of Love and Support?

After getting a life-threatening disease, when is a person more deserving of the love and support of others? Accept and embrace this love to help you heal. I have never interacted more, listened more, and learned from such a wide variety of people who generously shared their love and time with me. All of this love encouraged me to take better care of myself. During the times that I grew weary, this love became my impetus.

Make a list of the ways you can encourage and allow more love into your life and the ways you can embrace it, along with when you accepted and embraced the love of others.

_____

_____

_____

_____

_____

_____

_____

Write down every time you didn't, and why you turned your back on love. What did this cost you? How might you improve yourself?

_____

_____

_____

_____

_____

_____

_____

28

Don't Expect Yourself to Be Perfect— Be Compassionate with Yourself When You Make Mistakes

Before the Solaris blanket stopped the migraines, they had become intolerable. When I went for my annual checkup in 2014, I hoped my doctor would suggest something to help me. I was in no way prepared to hear I'd had a heart attack.

"Heart attack? No. Really? I don't think so. That makes no sense. I know my body. I'm sure I haven't."

"See this graph? This line should go up, but yours goes down, proving that you've had a heart attack. This is why you're feeling the pressure in your chest."

"You have no doubt whatsoever?"

"None."

"I think the pressure in my chest is from seeing how long I can hold a plank. I've been trying to strengthen my body hoping it might decrease the pain from the migraines."

"The test proves you've had a heart attack."

"The reason I even told you about this is because I know the pressure in the chest could be a side effect from Imitrex. I'm having migraines three to four times a week. Because they leave me exhausted, I've been trying to build up my physical strength before I become weak, and I turn into a blob of jello."

"It's a good thing you stopped taking the Imitrex because when you have a migraine, your blood vessels enlarge. The Imitrex works by making them smaller. Don't take the Imitrex anymore."

"But I'm still not convinced. Please stop and listen to me. What you're saying makes no sense."

"I'm recommending a good cardiologist for you. I'll ask her office to get in touch with you as soon as possible. Set up an appointment and see her right away. Don't put this off. And avoid exerting yourself. No more planks until after you've seen her."

"You sound so positive."

"This test proves you've had a heart attack."

"To think that I could be this wrong ... I thought I really knew my body. I can't believe I could be this far off. Does the test tell me when it happened?"

"The EKG only shows that you did."

"So, there's no doubt about this? I've definitely had a heart attack?"

"I have no doubt, so don't put this off. Get this checked right away. This is serious."

While driving out of the parking lot, I became light-headed. The fact that I had a heart attack and didn't know this ... I pulled my car over to the side of the road.

The way I'd taught myself to find safety in the world had just been blown to smithereens. I was living alone. I had little money, and the migraines had weakened my body, leaving me frail and vulnerable. I knew nothing about heart attacks other than they could kill you without warning. On some level, this reminded me of the AVM that could bleed and kill me in seconds.

I had developed an ability to know my body and this had given me security, but to now be told I no longer had this ... I called a friend. I planned to sound casual, but when I told him I had a heart attack, my voice cracked. I cried. He reminded me of the time a nurse had suspected I had one months before.

Did this mean my heart has been getting more and more damaged all this time?

Months earlier, while driving to work, as if I was watching a sci-fi movie, the fingers on my left hand slowly spiraled off the steering wheel on their own. Each finger twisted in a robotic fashion, one following the next like short little soldiers, until my hand was no longer grasping the wheel and fell onto my lap with a thump.

I'm having a heart attack, was my first thought and to call 911, but I didn't have any health insurance. Since the radiation had damaged the left side of my body, affecting my balance and hand, I told myself this was most likely the cause of this current problem. When it was out of my line of vision, my left hand would curl, my doctor had said, but I'd clearly seen it. My left hand had often curled, cupped on its own, though nothing like what I'd just seen.

Without any warning, again on its own, this hand lifted itself up from my lap and lightly grabbed the steering wheel, uncurling each finger in the opposite direction than it had less than a minute ago. Since I was close to the nursing home where I was working that day, I decided to wait and ask my favorite nurse for her opinion.

"You've had a heart attack. I'm calling 911 right now," she replied, and began walking briskly towards the nearest phone.

I yelled at her to stop, shouting that I had no health insurance and that I had yet to find a doctor who knew how to help me with the damage the radiation had caused. "I'll not get any help if you call 911 and I'll end up in debt for the rest of my life. Most of what I earn already goes to my healthcare."

"I would rather see you in debt than dead," she answered. "Wait. You work in the healthcare business and your company doesn't give you health insurance? Everyone knows how stressful working for hospice is."

"They know we love our patients."

"You're telling me that even though you work among some very sick people, you don't get paid sick days, and you're not given any health insurance? With a job like that, I can see why you'd have a heart attack."

I giggled. "Because I have a pre-existing condition, even if I could get insurance, the insurance company would say every problem I had was due to the brain tumor, and I'd have no way to prove it wasn't," I explained.

Just weeks before I was diagnosed with the heart attack, I received insurance from President Obama's Affordable Care Act. And my pre-existing condition no longer mattered. Thank you, Barack Obama!

Once home, I called a friend who told me about someone who had dropped dead from a heart attack. Assuming his nervousness had kept him from thinking about how this only added to my fears, I wondered how my estranged family would react if I suddenly died. I didn't want them to be surprised and feel guilty if I did. I wanted them to know I still loved them, so I emailed my mother and my two siblings.

I began each email by writing, "Don't be alarmed but ..." Neither my sister nor mother wrote back to me. Only my brother did.

"Don't be alarmed?! Well, if you're not alarmed, then you should be! I strongly hope you consult conventional medical expertise!" he wrote

I had been naïvely hoping he would thank me for thinking of him during this stressful time and would email me back something like, "I'm sorry this has happened to you." By this time, I had become used to people treating me kindly and respectfully. I had forgotten how my brother acted.

***

"I know you wouldn't want me criticizing anyone you love, but you need to face reality when it comes to your family," a friend later told me. "You can't keep expecting them to become different people, all warm and fuzzy and loving."

I had thought I'd learned to accept how my family acted, but it was evident that I hadn't, because my mother and sister's silence and my brother's email hit me hard. I had taken steps to accept them for who they were, but accepting that their need to protect themselves was greater than their love for me has been one of the hardest things I have ever done. To have to accept that they were so guarded that it prevented them from helping a close family member who had been diagnosed with a brain tumor, radiation damage and breast cancer, and now a heart attack, broke my heart.

One night, as I was watching a movie about the Unabomber, I felt his brother's pain when he realized how different his brother was from the way he had always seen him. When I finally was able to grasp the amount of anger, bitterness, and fear my family carried, I was devastated. My body grew weak. To help my body heal and for my peace of mind, I had to finally break this gut-wrenching habit and to see the members of my family as being who they are.

At least they're not making bombs and killing people, I thought, to keep myself from spiraling downward.

I had been told I had a heart attack on a Friday, before a three-day weekend, and to have it looked at right away. Since my doctor said not to exert myself, I stopped going to the gym and to work. As my anxiety heightened, my balance grew worse. No longer able to carry my laundry down two flights of stairs without possibly falling, dirty laundry mounted and my patience wore thin. Waiting for the cardiologist's office to call was torturous. When I could no longer wait, I called her office. I was told I had to wait six days to see the doctor.

171

My appointment began as usual with the doctor reviewing my health history until I got reprimanded, as if I were a child, for no longer seeing my oncologist.

"But he's the best," this tiny woman insisted twice after I told her the doctor's name. I tried to explain we simply thought differently, but she showed no interest in what I said. "But he's the best," she repeated for a third time.

Tired of this inappropriate treatment, I told this cardiologist that I had not come to discuss breast cancer with her. That I had been diagnosed as having a heart attack and I needed her help with this. She explained that the EKG test wasn't definite and told me to make another appointment on my way out so I could be tested the following week.

"But what about my chest pains?" I asked, and she told me to call 911 if they continued. Unhappy with the so-called care I was receiving, I drove myself to the emergency room when this pain continued the next day. After spending the night in the hospital, it was confirmed that I did indeed know my body because my heart tested stronger than 85 percent of people my age.

According to an article in *AARP: The Magazine*, the EKG test is known for its frequent misreadings. If a test comes back positive, *always* ask to have it retaken. Why my primary care doctor didn't know this, I'll never know.

If I hadn't been insured through the Affordable Care Act, this mistake would have cost me nearly $13,000. But the good news is (I do always look for the silver lining), I now am more confident than ever in my ability to know my body, and no doctor will ever fool me again.

Roll With the Punches

You must be resilient. People will disappoint you. Doctors will fall short of your expectations. Learning to play the best cards that you've been dealt is something you need to do. You'll often be dealt a losing hand that you have to make work. Stay present. Keep your heart open, stay in your body. In a somewhat similar way that you can feel the love of a loved one, feel the love in your heart encouraging you to go in a certain direction or to make a particular decision.

Make a list of the advantages you gained by being present and staying in your body, keeping your heart open and feeling love as it guided you.

_____

_____

_____

_____

_____

_____

_____

Make a list of the times you got stubborn and held onto your pain and aggravation, stayed in your head, and forgot to be more resilient and present and connected with your heart. And what did this cost you?

_____

_____

_____

_____

_____

_____

_____

29

Use Your Creativity to Assist Your Healing

People have frequently asked, "How can you be so positive after all you've been through?" I give much credit to doing art. Whether I'm facilitating an Expressive Arts workshop or creating art myself, art has brought love, joy, and healing into my life. It's given me a foundation and a way to ground myself, while it has also expanded my confidence and heart. It's no coincidence that creativity and our Creator have the same root word.

Expressive Art uses art in a therapeutic manner. Our attention is not on the piece of artwork itself. Here our focus is on the process of *doing* art. When we allow our hearts and our bodies' intuition to lead us, when we permit our hands to choose what colors to use, what kind of marks to make, and how to make them, buried treasures from within our bodies become unearthed.

Doing Expressive Art reminds us that our strength is inside us. It's become popular today, and is used in hospitals, nursing homes, hospices, cancer centers, mental health facilities, churches, schools, and many other facilities and homes all over the world, because those who do Expressive Art can access and feel their inner strength. And from this, they heal. Plus, it's fun and the rewards are endless because it assists each person in the way they need.

It helps us heal by releasing past negative experiences and the false beliefs that we all carry in our bodies. Things we might not even know exist, or have the ability to express in words, can be accessed by connecting to the sacred, silent, peaceful place inside us and be freed from our bodies when using Expressive Art.

While I was working as an Expressive Art Specialist for hospice, my job was to help patients find comfort by connecting to this strength within. This helped the patients' passing go as smoothly and pain-free as possible.

When I met a new patient, I would first determine what she enjoyed. Agatha told me she missed seeing the bluebirds that flew in her backyard and that she liked to color. Every time I visited her, I drew bluebirds (because she couldn't) that she would then color. Similar to a string of paper dolls, I attached these birds to long pieces of string, which I fastened to the ceiling and strung across her room.

"I used to sit with my bluebirds outside, but now I get to sleep among them," she told me, while smiling during our last visit.

Mary missed walking and seeing the sights in her neighborhood, so I walked around her block and took photographs. I attached each of these photos to foam board and held each one above her head as she lay in her bed. Together we "walked" through her neighborhood as she smiled, delighted she got to see her old familiar sights again.

Doing Expressive Art increased the patients' comfort. As they became more comfortable, their resistance softened, and they became more receptive to their medical care. Their trust and happiness increased, which contributed to their ability to have loving and fulfilling relationships and find enjoyment in their lives.

Our immune systems work more efficiently when our spirits rise and our stress levels decrease. This "branch of medicine that deals with the influence of emotional states, such as stress and happiness, and how our nervous systems affect our immune function, especially in relation to the onset and progression of disease," is called psychoneuroimmunology, as defined by the Merriam-Webster dictionary.

A hospice patient "graduates" when her health is no longer declining. While I don't have statistics to back this up (because, to the best of my knowledge, none yet exist), I noted a high percentage of my patients lived much longer than just six months, and many of them graduated.

We benefit whenever we slow down and follow where our bodies lead, when we don't let our heads and fears be our guides. Expressive Art is a useful and fun tool, and it helps us live in the present moment. It stops the harmful habit of believing that the answers to our problems are outside of us. Expressive Art also helps us to become more intuitive. The more we practice Expressive Art, the stronger our instincts grow and the easier it is to access our inner voice. The more we trust our instincts, the better decisions we make healthwise and in every way.

For the first 40 years of my life, I had never heard the term "Expressive Art," though I unknowingly practiced it. Since my experience in the winter of 1987, when I was shocked to discover that death was a theme in my art, Expressive Art has become popular with artists, therapists, theologians, and others, because it helps us to better understand our authentic selves and heal.

Expressive Art "awakens the Holy that resides within," wrote Pastor Rebecca Bradburn Langer, D. Min., Adjunct Faculty, San Francisco Theological Seminary Program in Christian Spirituality.

It's also been called the language of the soul because it allows us "to have a conversation and communion with the One," wrote Jan Richardson, artist and author of *In Wisdom's Path: Discovering the Sacred in Every Season*.

In 1993, I painted the mural because my body told me I had to share what I learned to help others and to celebrate my life. And I knew to trust this. From among the thousands who came to see it, two women stepped forward from the crowd: Barbara Ganim and Susan Fox. Barbara asked to interview me for a book she was writing on Expressive Art.

"Sure," I replied. "But what's Expressive Art?"

Silence followed as these women looked at each other until Susan said, "You just did it in a big way!"

Both women taught Expressive Art at Salve Regina University in Newport, RI, less than an hour from where I lived. I studied with them both and became a certified Expressive Art facilitator.

"This longing to reflect an inner vision or give form to feelings allows us to travel on a more meaningful inner journey. It's an exploration of the heart," wrote Susan, who is now the author of several books, as is Barbara who wrote *Art and Healing: Using Expressive Art to Heal Your Body, Mind and Spirit*.

Barbara Ganim wrote "The immune system—our inner power source of healing and wellness—is suppressed by stress-producing negative thoughts, unresolved emotions, anger, anxiety, and fear. Our verbal thoughts keep our bodies in a state of stress most of the time. When our imagery, expressed through some form of art, is focused on sending a soothing, stress-releasing message to the body, the immune system is freed to activate the healing process. When art is used on a regular basis, we will begin to live lives of inner peace and harmony—the keys to long-term healing."

Was it just a coincidence that I never stopped doing art as most adults do? Did I major in art in college knowing on some unconscious level that I needed art to help heal me? Of course, I have no way of knowing, but if you feel the desire to be creative in any way, I suggest you never hold yourself back, thinking you're not good enough.

Find Fun and Creative Ways to Help Yourself Heal

If our immune systems become "suppressed by stress-producing negative thoughts, unresolved emotions, anger, anxiety, and fear," as Barbara Ganim wrote, in what ways can you help yourself heal? Whenever you think negative thoughts, stop yourself—but don't become a Pollyanna. We all need to vent and complain at times and express our needs. Whenever you hear yourself complaining about anything, change your focus to finding the solution. Bring creativity into your life: painting, dancing, singing, writing poetry, cooking, doing origami, photography, or making jewelry, to name just a few of many ways.

Make a list of the ways you can bring creativity into your life to assist your healing.

_____

_____

_____

_____

_____

_____

Write down every time you just complained and didn't look for the solution. Notice when you're having negative thoughts that are working against you. And why have you not pursued a creative outlet?

_____

_____

_____

_____

_____

_____

_____

30

What a Helpful Article for All!

I was thrilled when I discovered an article titled, "How Not to Say the Wrong Thing," written by Susan Silk and Barry Goldman for the *L.A. Times*.

When Susan was recuperating from surgery, she told a colleague she wasn't up to having visitors.

"This isn't about you," the colleague replied.

Who else this could be about? Susan wondered until she realized her colleague thought *her* desires took precedence. After a similar thing happened a second time, Susan found a way to protect the sick and vulnerable by developing a technique she calls "The Ring Theory." I think it's ingenious.

You begin by drawing a small center ring. The name of the person who has a trauma goes inside this. For example, after I got sick, my name would have been written in this center ring.

The person in the center ring may have been traumatized by an illness, the death of a loved one, going to war, maybe losing a job—any kind of trauma. She is allowed to say to anyone at any time anything she wants. She can cry, scream, and even curse God without any resistance or shaming from anyone. In other words, to assist with her healing, she is not to be restricted from expressing herself in any way.

You then draw a second circle around the first and write the names of the people who are closest to the person in the center circle. Since my mother was closest to me, she would have been in the next circle, so she could complain to my siblings, but not to me. My siblings would have been in the next circle, so their responsibility was to support my mother and me, and not complain to either of us. What a help it would have been if I had been shielded in this way! My life would not have been as difficult or been filled with so much sadness and confusion.

One thing I love about "The Ring Theory" is that everyone gets the opportunity to express themselves. Anyone can say whatever they want, but only to people in a larger ring. I cannot emphasize enough how important it is that no one feels invisible or silenced.

Susan also explains that it's far more important to listen than to talk and to only talk to those in smaller circles, if what you say is comforting and supportive. She wrote that most people know not to be critical of the person in the center ring, and I agree—which is why I was so shocked when I discovered my own family didn't know this.

To make it easier to remember how "The Ring Theory" works, Susan suggested people simply remember "comfort in", meaning to comfort those in the smaller rings and "dump out," complain only to those in the larger rings.

It was because my family was so angry with me that I began an intensive study on human behavior. Originally, I didn't plan to include my family in this book, but so that readers could learn from my experience, I had to include how their behavior affected my healing and how I coped with this. By understanding why some people might react in a cruel and hurtful way after you are diagnosed with a life-threatening illness, I hope readers will be prepared to avoid this pain and confusion that could compromise their health.

I knew that the members of my family enjoyed being comforted when they were sick, and that being screamed at and shamed would make them feel worse, so for years, their peculiar behavior baffled me. Despite attending 12-step meetings for adult children of alcoholics for 13 years, I never knew a family addiction could affect someone with a terminal illness in such a detrimental and significant way.

In her article, Susan wrote that "The Ring Theory" merely "expands our intuition and makes it more concrete." When I read this, my stomach clenched. The members in my family had been taught to avoid what they felt, so "The Ring Theory" wouldn't "expand their intuition and make it more concrete." They kept themselves from knowing what most people intuitively knew.

On the other hand, the members of my family were extraordinarily adaptable. They learned to hide their deficiencies behind their charming personalities, intelligence, good looks, and sense of humor. Their smoke screens were so impressive that until I got sick and needed their help, I had no idea how emotionally handicapped and dysfunctional they were.

If I could wave a magic wand, what would I have wanted? To be supported by my loving family so that I felt safe and protected. This would have alleviated much stress on me, as opposed to contributing to it. If my family had listened and allowed me to express myself, I would not have thought I was as damaged as I did for years.

I have pictured myself in the center ring, protected, not afraid to cry or say anything, and having my fears and needs heard and respected. I can only imagine what it would be like if I had not been judged and ridiculed. If I hadn't been treated like a leper, my life would have been so different.

No one gets to decide when a toddler takes his first step. A toddler gets up and walks according to when his body is ready. If my family had supported me to heal the way my body chose and at its own pace, my healing would not have taken so long and been so challenging. A toddler needs to feel safe before he attempts to walk. Being pushed before he's ready, criticizing and trying to take this control from him, is counterproductive. I believe my siblings deserve to heal from their pain and anger in their own way and at their own pace, just as everyone does—including me.

There were times when I resented my family because of my struggle and pain due to this additional stress on my weary body. But then I remembered that the members of my family were simply being who they are, and like everyone else, they had every right to be wherever they were on their life's journey. And that I had to take responsibility for the part I played.

I loved and still love my family. I have always wanted them to be in my life. For decades, not for one second, was I willing to give up on them. I had unwavering faith and believed that they would become capable of seeing their behavior and that how they treated me was reprehensible. I had hoped for a long time that they would have wanted to take responsibility for their actions, learn and grow from their experience.

I have never wanted to live without my family. I could have written them off long ago and decided they were insensitive jerks. I could have gone about my life free from their incessant need for the ongoing drama they created in my life at the worst possible time.

Once I taught myself to focus on the love I had in my life, and not on the love of my family that I missed, my life aligned around this mindset and my healing accelerated.

Expanding Your Thinking, Changing Your Habits

Expand your thinking and understanding about people. You have to accept their deficits. In this stress-filled world, more people are living in a state of continual stress, making it impossible for them to think beyond their own needs. Their survival instincts are so severe, their thinking so restricted and distorted, that they can't even recognize that someone with a life-threatening disease needs their support.

Make a list of the ways you have accepted how other people behave. Notice what a life-changing, stress-reducing tool this is.

_____

_____

_____

_____

_____

_____

_____

_____

Notice how often you haven't been able to accept how other people behave and you couldn't accept their behavior. Write down the stress this caused you and any other costs.

_____

_____

_____

_____

_____

_____

_____

_____

31

Life Continues Regardless of Your Circumstances

In the winter of 2017, my mother's caregiver found her lying unconscious on the dining room floor, cold to the touch but still breathing. After being rushed to the hospital, it was quickly assessed that she had overdosed. She spent the next 30 days rehabilitating. Now, having hardly recognized her for the past three decades, I finally got glimpses of the mother I once knew. There were a few moments when we appreciated each other and laughed together on the phone, just like we used to do.

For years, she had been hurling angry jabs at me, but now this stopped. I took advantage of this time to tell her I had long forgiven her for hurting me, and that I hoped she had forgiven me, too, though my words were followed by silence. I suspect this may have been too intimate a conversation for her. I told her how much I appreciated how our love had held us together all these years. Again, she said nothing, but I got to express my love for her.

Because I attended 12-step meetings for 13 years, and was close friends with Gainor, who was a recovering alcoholic, I knew permanent health issues and even death could occur when someone was withdrawing from an addiction; that this was why withdrawals needed to be done in a reputable medical facility that specialized in addictions. Depending on the severity of the addiction, seizures, tremors, heart attacks, and strokes could occur. My mother's addiction was unquestionably severe. Although she sounded good when we spoke, I was still worried about her because I questioned the competence of the facility where she'd gone to rehabilitate.

I had lived with my mother's lies and manipulation during the most vulnerable time in my life, so I understood why my sister had become frustrated living close to her and why she had called me frequently to vent. After hearing how resentful and unraveled my sister had become, there came a time when I didn't know who was worse off: my mother or my sister.

Al-Anon exists to help the loved ones of addicts cope with the addict's nerve-wracking behavior. It teaches people how to protect themselves and learn effective protective techniques. I had suggested to my sister more than once that she attend Al-Anon to learn the skills I'd learned because I knew it would help her, but she showed no interest.

"I'm not getting involved. Mom is an adult and can make her own decisions," she told me, to which I replied that Mom wasn't the one I was worried about.

I'm guessing that my sister and mother didn't know the importance of having Mom's withdrawal overseen at a skilled rehabilitation center. However, they both knew that I knew more about addictions than either of them. But the decision as to where my mother went for rehabilitation was made without asking my opinion.

My mother chose to go to a rehabilitation center where she had been twice before, once when she fell and once when she was malnourished. When her 30-day rehabilitation ended, since she could no longer live alone, she moved into the same facility's long-term housing section.

Days later, just as I feared, she had a stroke. I have no idea why 12 hours passed before an ambulance was called, and why no one on the staff noticed she was having problems sooner. After my mother was discharged from the hospital, my sister called and told me, "It's a miracle that Mom is alive!" I kept my suspicions to myself and wasn't surprised when my sister called back a few days later to tell me, "Mom's doctor suggested I call hospice."

"Knowing that Mom will get the best care possible from hospice makes hearing this easier," was the first thing I said.

"Her heart has been badly damaged. She's slowly dying. Days. Maybe weeks. Her doctor couldn't say, so you don't have to rush down to Florida to be by her side. Take your time," my sister said in a soft quivering voice.

I was thinking that my suspicions were probably right. My mother should have gone to a facility that specialized in substance abuse, but it was too late now. My mother had been insistent about where she wanted her rehabilitation to occur.

Allow your love to strengthen you, Sandi. Keep your heart open. I knew nothing more could be done for my mother, so I focused on supporting my sister. As our mother's health declined, she did her best to assist her, but caring for someone with health problems came no easier to her than it had to our mother.

"I got stuck looking after Mom because she lived so close, not because of her love for me, but because she loves my two boys," my sister had once said.

"I'm glad Mom's doctor knew to suggest hospice," I told her, concerned that she sounded so frail. "Hospice also specializes in helping the families during this time. This will make things easier for all of us. After Mom dies, you'll never have to second-guess yourself, wonder if you made the right choices, or did enough."

God knows my poor sister doesn't need to be saddled with this.

"Hospice will be a huge help to you. When it comes to helping the dying, they know more than nursing homes do, which is the reason they exist. Otherwise, there'd be no need. They'll take this pressure off you and—"

An ear-piercing scream cut me off. Someone was in excruciating pain. Shaken by this, I asked, "What the hell was that?"

"Oh. That's Mom. She screams like she's having a baby every time she's flipped, whenever they change her. I should have left her room before calling you," my sister said, sounding much too casual.

"What?! That's Mom screaming? That's not right. She shouldn't be suffering at all. Why hasn't she been given painkillers?"

"She's been given painkillers," my sister replied, sighing loudly into the phone.

I suspect she wanted to let me know how annoying I was for having the nerve to be concerned about our mother being in pain. Believing her stress must be affecting her judgement, I paused before I gently said, "Please think about this. Mom wouldn't be screaming if she had enough painkillers. Right? Doesn't that make sense?"

A few years before, my mother told me that because my sister lived near her, my sister would make the decisions regarding her health care when she was no longer able. I assured my mother that I understood and would respect her wishes, though I thought I wouldn't want my sister making these decisions for me.

After our phone call ended, I was sad, but also happy I didn't add to her stress by getting emotional. I felt pleased that even under these circumstances I was able to think of her and offer what help I could. I wondered if my sister noticed and would appreciate how I treated her.

I had never felt more grateful that I'd worked for hospice. My sister knew I had years of experience with end-of-life care. I knew this would take a lot of pressure off her. And this felt good.

After we talked, I was so sure my mother's pain would end in minutes that I never gave this another thought. I found comfort knowing that hospice would soon be helping both my mother and sister, just as I had seen hospice often do for others. I was sure by the time I arrived in Florida, this heavy burden would be lifted from my sister's shoulders, and my mother would pass peacefully.

All that night I couldn't stop my mind from racing. I kept wondering if my mother's heart wouldn't have been damaged had she gone to a facility that specialized in drug withdrawal. While I was tossing and turning, I decided to keep my suspicions to myself because there was no point in upsetting my siblings. Plus, I couldn't prove it, anyway.

I was cat-sitting for a friend, so I couldn't immediately leave. This allowed me to get some much-needed rest before going to the Providence airport, taking two planes, renting a car, and driving for over an hour to my sister's home. Never had I traveled this much since I'd first been diagnosed with the brain tumor.

I arrived exhausted at my sister's home ready to go to bed, but my sister had other plans. Just minutes after my arrival, looking stiff, nervous, and avoiding eye contact, she announced that she had made a decision. A social worker at the facility where our mother was staying had suggested that hospice not be called unless our mother was still alive at the end of the week. And my sister had agreed with this.

Fear shot through my body. I was scared for my mother, scared for my sister, scared of what the days ahead might bring. Being as exhausted as I was, I just kept a poker face and went to bed. But my mind was racing.

Connect with the love within for strength.

My sister had taken advice from the social worker who was being paid by this facility, instead of taking the advice of Mom's doctor! And this made sense to her? Had she not realized that this was to the facility's advantage and may not be to Mom's? Her doctor had suggested that hospice be called because *they* specialized in end-of-life care. Didn't this mean anything to her?

She knew I worked for hospice, and yet she had made this decision knowing I would soon arrive. And she offered no explanation other than that it was easier. And why would she make this decision on her own when she knew this was a family matter?

Most families unite during such a sensitive time and discuss these issues among themselves—unless they are dysfunctional. Oh. This would explain why she was acting like she was an only child. Having control had always given her a sense of security.

I already had my suspicions about the care this facility offered. If what I feared was about to happen ... I prayed my sister could forgive herself for going against Mom's doctor's advice. All she had to do was wait for me before making this decision, but she chose to take this entirely on herself. Why was she sabotaging herself and risking Mom's care? She obviously didn't care about what I thought.

"Hospice has a reputation of over-drugging their patients," she told me the next day while driving, and she could avoid eye contact.

Meaning she made this decision based on rumors and fear. Without asking for my opinion, she had chosen to just believe this. Was not hiring hospice giving her a feeling of control that she craved? But what about later, years from now? How would she feel about her decision then?

I prayed, for Mom and my sister's sake, that going against the doctor would turn out the way my sister wanted and, if it didn't, she wouldn't allow her guilt to consume her. If she was unable to accept responsibility for her choice, she had better not blame Mom or me for these problems she'd brought on herself. Then again, knowing her, she would have to blame someone. And with Mom gone, that would be me, no doubt.

Unable to sleep, as soon as I heard birds chirping the next morning, I got out of bed to go see my mother. As was common in Florida, the facility where she was staying offered everything from drug rehabilitation to assisted living, inpatient and outpatient care, long-term living, and rehabilitation after surgeries, much like "one-stop shopping," which as most people know, always came at a cost.

As I drove into the parking lot, I was surprised to see my thin-haired brother standing next to a large palm tree. His head was lowered to his chest. His belly was protruding. At first, I didn't recognize him. He looked so old and frail. I called his name as I got out of my car and watched as his head snapped up. Immediately, he raised his chin in an unsuccessful attempt to look confident, a telltale sign which meant he wasn't.

"Mom hasn't spoken in two days, so don't expect her to say anything. It's really bad," he warned me as we were about to enter our mother's room.

When she saw me, her eyes lit up, and she smiled widely. Using her skinny arms and elbows, she strained to raise herself up from the bed to offer me a proper greeting. When I saw how weak she was, my heart felt like it was being torn from my chest, though I was delighted to see how happy she was to see me. To have this opportunity to feel my mother's love again ... I kissed her on her cheek and sat down on her bed, held her hand. As tears streamed down my face, I told her how much I loved her.

I went into my hospice mode. Some of the facilities where I'd worked had failed to keep their patients hydrated, so I asked my mother if she was thirsty. She nodded yes. I found some lip balm on the small table next to her bed and moistened her dry lips before holding a glass of water gently against them.

I was appalled to see how thirsty she was. I had never seen a patient this dehydrated. I felt awful for my mother and utter disgust for this place. After she laid back down, I gently stroked her forehead with a cool, moist cloth, hoping the care she was receiving would prove to be better than I'd just witnessed.

"I love you, Mom. Tell me what I can do for you. You know I'll do anything for you. Just tell me and I'll do it," I promised through tears.

She strained to lift her head again. I leaned down close to her.

"Make it stop," she whispered.

Make what stop? End her life? No, she's asking me to stop her pain. "Stop your pain?" I asked, and she nodded. She smiled, while looking relieved, fell back down onto her pillow and closed her eyes.

Years before, my mother asked me how I could work for hospice.

"I wouldn't be able to do my job if, whenever I had a patient so much as grimace in pain, I couldn't ask that more medication be given."

Because dying is difficult enough without being painful too, most patient's doctors prescribed high dosages of painkillers, in case more was needed. Unlike what my sister believed, hospice doesn't over-medicate their patients. Since all medications are regulated by the Federal Food and Drug Administration, hospice is only authorized to follow what each patient's doctor has prescribed.

When I worked for hospice, I never once saw a patient suffer. Everyone was treated with respect and dignity. This is what I was used to seeing. Years before, I told my mother if I had to watch anyone suffer, I would have had to quit my job. So my mother knew while she was dying that I would have done whatever it took to make sure she wasn't in pain. I was glad my brother had been there, watching our interaction. He saw how comfortable I was in this environment and that I knew what I was doing.

"I thought we'd lost her two days ago. She hadn't spoken since, but she responded to you. I feel like I'd just witnessed a miracle."

I smiled and said, "You did. It's called love."

I closed my eyes and deeply inhaled this family-united-wonderful-feeling, something I hadn't felt and had painfully missed for over 20 years. I extended the love I felt to include my brother. Silently, I thanked God for giving me this opportunity to experience my mother's love again and that my brother had been here to witness and share this.

Two nurse's assistants came into the room to change my mother, and we promptly exited.

There's a Reason 12-Step Meetings and Counselors Exist

If you are emotionally struggling, get the help you need and deserve. If you want to heal and you want the world to be a more loving place, and you're not contributing to this, get the help you need.

Make a list of why you would want to be a loving contributor and ways you could create more love in your life and subsequently, the world.

_____

_____

_____

_____

_____

_____

_____

_____

_____

List the ways you're holding yourself back, and why. What is this costing you? And if you *are* holding yourself back, why?

_____

_____

_____

_____

_____

_____

_____

_____

_____

32

Notice How Much You've Grown

As my brother and I stepped into the hallway, our sister was walking towards us down a long corridor. I felt sad to see her looking so taut and skeletal. Her eyes were dark and sunken. Did she really suffer from anorexia as Gainor once suggested?

"Anorexia is common in Adult Children of Alcoholics. You know, you guys can be just as messed up as us alcoholics, sometimes even more," she'd said while laughing.

Still feeling elated from my mother's love, I excitedly greeted my sister. I was telling her about Mom greeting me when agonizing screams penetrated through Mom's door. I can only imagine the expression on my face when I realized my mother was still in pain and her suffering hadn't ended.

"Mom's been in pain all this time?!" I asked. My siblings continued to talk with one another as if they hadn't heard anything. "Mom's still in pain?!" I shouted.

Slowly, my brother and sister turned to look at me with blank expressions on their faces.

"Nothing's been done to stop Mom's pain?!" I asked.

Only silence followed.

"You have got to be kidding me! Why hasn't Mom been given enough painkillers to stop her pain?" I asked and waited for an answer. When it was clear that my question was being ignored, I took off running to the nearest nurse's station. Here I was told that "it would be looked into" while I wondered what the hell was wrong with this place.

When I returned to my mother's room and asked my sister why Mom's pain continued, she offered to give me a tour of the facility. To show me how professional they were? Did she hope I would be convinced to trust this awful place?

As we roamed the hallways together, my sister held her chin up high, avoided eye contact, and smugly smiled. I could see that having faith in this facility gave her comfort. I had to tread carefully, so I told her how beautiful the facility was. And it was. But to me it was obvious that they were using this fancy façade to attract naïve customers.

My sister beamed at my compliment, as if she owned the place, and shared her plan to bring the staff platters of food "after," to show her appreciation for all their help. She especially liked their social worker who had gone out of her way to assist her.

For all the help they've given you? What about Mom, who's been screaming in pain for days? Why isn't their attention on Mom's comfort? Why isn't yours? I wanted to yell, but didn't.

Despite knowing that our mother had been screaming in pain for at least four days that I knew of, my sister was pleased with this facility. No wonder Mom had woken up and asked for my help.

My family had always been good at avoiding what we didn't want to see and believing only what we wanted to believe, just like I had done by only seeing the best in my family when I was young as my survival tactic.

I noticed that my sister said "after," and not "after Mom dies." Did this mean that the person in charge of deciding the best care for Mom still did not accept that Mom was dying?

"I keep asking myself what would happen if I took Mom home. What if we're already needlessly overmedicating her? Have you thought about this, Sandi?"

I looked at my sister with sympathy and fear.

"But then I remember what the doctor said about her failing heart ... and all the tests she had ... I guess I really have to believe she's never going to leave this place like she always had every other time I've brought her here."

My sister had lived for years in fear of our mother overdosing, just as I had, so I knew how tough this was. Because she was the one who was called every time our mother did, this had to have been even worse for her.

Was she not allowing Mom to have more painkillers because she was afraid she would overdose again? Is the reason she wouldn't hire hospice because she feared they would overmedicate Mom and kill her?

My sister could hear Mom screaming just as loudly as I could. Is it possible that she found Mom's screams comforting because as long as she heard them, this meant that Mom was still alive?

How I wished my sister had gone to 12-step meetings where she would have learned how to cope with our mother having a drug addiction. But the problem was she thought she could. Had she been more self-aware, Mom's dying would have been easier on her and all of us.

While we toured the facility, I told my sister that, except in rare cases, no one had to ever die in pain. She responded by pointing out how surprised she was to see that half of the beds were empty in the rooms we walked by. She said she had never seen the facility this empty in all the years she had been bringing Mom here.

I don't know what my sister thought about these beds being empty, or if she thought about it at all, but I associated empty beds with loss of money. I wondered if, to make up for this facility's financial loss, this social worker had taken advantage of my sister's vulnerability.

The next day, the two of us were sitting by our mother's bedside, exhausted by our grief. The social worker, this woman my sister adored, didn't even ask us how we were before she told us a long story about washing her cat the night before, and its underarm hair getting tangled in its armpits.

"The groomer charged me $400!" she whined as my sister and I sat grieving for our dying mother.

We were about to enter a foreign, dreaded, and grueling world. After becoming motherless, our lives would never be the same. We both stared at this woman in disbelief. She must have realized her mistake because she stopped her jabbering and quickly left the room.

"That was totally inappropriate," I whispered to my sister on the other side of our mother's bed.

"I guess," she could barely say.

My sister had just been forced to see how self-serving and unprofessional this woman was—this person, whose advice she had taken regarding our mother's care. *How will she handle this? Will she be able to?* I didn't want her blaming herself or feeling guilty so I said, "You made the best decision you could, with the tools you had."

"Yes, with the tools I had," she said, staring off into space.

As much as I wanted to know what she was thinking, seeing how emotionally flooded she was, I wasn't about to fulfill my own desires and put more pressure on her.

If only my sister had waited and asked for my opinion before making her final decision, she wouldn't be feeling all this pressure on her. Had she been willing to appreciate or respect my advice and included me, since I was experienced with end-of-life care, she wouldn't be in the fragile shape she was in now.

Was she even capable of understanding what this revealed about the social worker and the care our mother was receiving? Would she have to pretend this never happened? As we sat with our dying mother on the bed between us, I tried my best to support her, knowing this was the most loving thing I could do for my poor sister.

"Remember, you've never had a mother die before. I know you're doing the best you can, so try not to beat yourself up."

Before I flew to Florida, I made it my goal to accomplish two things: to do all I could to help my mother's transition to be as comfortable as possible, and to support my siblings through this difficult time. My plan was to be as supportive as I could be, while also respecting my own grief and needs.

My hope was that we would grow closer by sharing this time together. After all, our original four-member family was about to become three.

What added to my frustration is that neither of my siblings ever seemed to learn and grow from their challenges. I was hoping I would be surprised by the changes in them, but when I got to Florida, they showed no signs of maturing, and the protective walls around them hadn't softened at all.

Did they notice that I was mourning our mother's passing too, and that I was doing this on my own? Did they ever wonder what it had been like as a single woman who had no kids to be separated and ostracized by the only family I had?

I never stopped asking that more painkillers be given. Only after three long, difficult, and miserable days was morphine finally given. But whenever my mother was turned in her bed, she still screamed in agony.

Since she had been in this same facility for her 30-day drug rehabilitation, had just been treated for drug abuse less than two weeks before, how was it possible that no one here knew what drugs were needed to manage her pain?

When I asked that more morphine be given, a nurse looked at me with a puzzled look on her face and said, "We've given her enough to drop a horse. I honestly don't understand."

***

"Every patient I saw when I worked for hospice rested comfortably on inflatable mattresses, so they didn't have to be turned and disrupted," I told my sister. "If they can't reduce Mom's pain, would you please ask that they stop turning Mom or get an air mattress?"

"Will you?" my sister asked, now wanting my help.

"They know you and that you're in charge. There's a far better chance they will listen to you."

A short while later, the head of nursing came into my mother's room where I was sitting alone beside my mother. "I heard you're not happy with the care your mother's receiving," she said.

Feeling sad and depleted, I said, "My mother has been screaming in pain and she asked me to stop it. This is the last thing my mother will ever say to me. There's no way anyone can stop me from fulfilling her last wishes, so please don't try to stop me or this could get ugly, which is the last thing I want."

"But she needs to be turned or she'll get bedsores."

"So, either give her enough pain medication so she'll stop screaming whenever she's turned, or provide a proper inflatable air mattress. Either way is fine with me. I've worked for hospice, and I know dying patients should never have to suffer like this."

"We really shouldn't be having this conversation in front of your mother."

"Then why did you start it here? Surely, you know I didn't."

It felt like my mother was listening, cheering me on, but I agreed to step into one of the empty rooms across the hall. Here I explained my health history to this nurse, so she knew I was experienced with medical care. I told her my only agenda was to make sure my mother died with the peace and dignity that she deserved.

"I understand and admire your love and dedication to your mother."

"And I appreciate that someone is finally listening to me after four long, torturous days."

"Since hospice will be here in two days, I'll see to it that your mother is no longer turned. And I shouldn't be telling you this, but I agree with you. I think how you think."

"Thank you for sharing that."

"Once your mother passes, I have no doubt your siblings will recognize and appreciate the love and dedication you've shown. Your courage to speak up is admirable."

***

So that she wouldn't have to wonder and have additional stress on her, I had told my sister when I first arrived in Florida that I knew Mom had put her in charge and I would support her. Yet just a day later, I had to remind her that it was important that we both respected Mom's wishes—that Mom put her in charge of her healthcare but Mom asked me to stop her pain. I thought she understood this, until hours later she became belligerent.

I was sitting alone by my mother's bedside holding her hand when my sister entered the room. Standing about ten feet from me, she said, "I know you think I enjoy watching Mom suffer."

I looked at her in disbelief. Refusing to add to her stress and trauma, I took a breath and calmly replied, "I've been nothing but supportive of you the entire time I've been here. And you know this, right?"

I paused and smiled warmly, to give her a moment to think while I focused on the love in my heart to give myself strength. While waiting for my sister to answer, silently I sent her love.

When all I got back was silence, I continued, "I've respectfully acquiesced to all your decisions, haven't I? And I told you I appreciate you looking after Mom when she got old, and that I understand why letting her go must be difficult for you in particular."

And still she said nothing. Just stared at me.

"Mom made a request of me as well. Not just you. Do you really think it would be right if I were to ignore this?"

I paused again and waited.

"Just like I've been respecting what Mom asked of you, you need to respect what Mom asked of me, too. You can make this all about you, but Mom is dying and in pain. Why would you think I'm thinking about you? Surely, you can see that my hands have been full, trying to get her pain to end."

I waited and hoped she would appreciate the love and patience I was showing her. But she said nothing before exiting the room. Sharing our mother like this must have been too challenging for her, when she wasn't used to it.

My sister never learned to ground and nurture herself, so she believed others created her problems. This was the same self-destructive pattern that hadn't changed since childhood. This is why she grew older, but never wiser. And why she never found peace within herself.

She had to have seen how I reacted to her ugly accusation while I was also exhausted from grieving. She couldn't deny that I responded to her with love, could she? I had been watching her use this hit-and-run tactic in reaction to conflict since she was a child, lashing out like a snake when she felt threatened, before slithering away and exiting a room.

Accusing, avoiding, and refusing to take responsibility for her actions is exactly what our mother did too. As an adult, my sister never learned effective ways to cope with stress. No wonder the poor woman had grown so frail and bitter.

I had tried to include her and my entire family in my healing journey. My hope had been that we all could have grown together and benefited from the pain we each experienced. But the three of them fought me tooth and nail. Even while our mother was dying, this continued. Because none of them was willing to look at their own behavior and take responsibility for it, nothing changed. Thankfully, I did.

"You gain strength, courage, and confidence by every experience in which you stop to look fear in the face. You must do the thing you think you cannot do," Eleanor Roosevelt said.

My family refused to look fear in the face, or perhaps they didn't have the courage or see the need. Instead, they chose to blame me for their fears and discomfort, and so they lost their opportunity to learn and grow.

Just hours after my sister's sneak attack, my brother and his wife entered Mom's room where my sister and I were sitting. As he walked in, his chin was raised, displaying this same old telltale family trait that revealed he was emotionally struggling, but pretending not to be. Before he said hello, he announced that the staff wasn't happy because "my two sisters have insisted on telling them how to do their jobs."

How was it even possible that he believed I cared more about what the staff thought than stopping Mom's pain?

He instructed my sister and I to step into the hall.

"You just sell things on eBay that you find in thrift stores and yet you think you have the right to tell these professionals how to do their jobs?" he said to me, before turning to our sister. "And you're just a housewife and you're now questioning these professionals, too?"

I had noticed earlier that my brother never sat by our mother's bed. Like clockwork, once in the morning and once in the afternoon, he stood, walked over to where Mom was lying, and placed one hand over hers. He whispered something for a minute or two before he retreated to his wife's side in a section of the room farthest from our mother.

Since I knew how emotions challenged him, I had been feeling sorry for him, wondering how he would cope with Mom's dying. He had just demonstrated how: by attempting to control and shame his two grieving sisters.

We had all gone out to dinner the night before. Taking advantage of the warm Florida weather, we sat outside around a large wooden picnic table and shared family memories. I had been quiet, enjoying this walk down memory lane, until my brother announced that he had decided when he was young that he was a genius when he realized he was smarter than his two sisters.

Much like the jarring loud buzzer sound that announces halftime at a basketball game, my whole body reacted to his words with a jolt, before I intellectually understood. Putting us down was my brother's way of attempting to find comfort for himself.

Keep your heart open. He's having a tough time. Send him some supportive love.

Respect People Who Think Differently Than You.
Accept That They Have the Right To.

I viewed the medical care my mother was receiving differently from my siblings, but I didn't try to convince them to think like me or get angry at them. How I thought upset them and they both tried to change me, which added to their pain and misery. I viewed the facility as incompetent, while my siblings trusted and probably found security and comfort in trusting the medical center's professionalism. We can't expect everyone to think like us.

Make a list of the times you accepted that someone thought differently than you did. What are the advantages of accepting that others will think differently?

_____

_____

_____

_____

_____

_____

Can you see how expecting others to think like you is as futile as expecting everyone to have your color hair? Can you see that thinking everyone should think like you creates stress in your life?

List the times thinking like this has caused you problems. And what is the cost to you and your relationships?

_____

_____

_____

_____

_____

_____

33

You Are Stronger Than You Think

It was clear my brother's goal was not to be supportive of me or my sister as we grieved for our dying mother together. The strain on his face was evident, but I couldn't afford to be used as his punching bag. I was not about to yell back at him and add to his misery, so I held my hand up like a traffic cop, gesturing for him to stop.

"No one has the right to talk to me like that," I said with poise and dignity, and turned to rejoin my dying mother.

Has he never learned that treating people in this arrogant manner won't bring him the comfort he seeks? Don't either of my siblings know not to yell at someone who's grieving for their dying mother? How sad is this?

As badly as I felt for the two of them, I also felt a sense of satisfaction: even under these grueling circumstances, I remained grounded in love. Despite my two siblings attacking me, I had acted more mature than both of them. After feeling degraded and guilty for having a temper for years, I now felt grateful for all I'd learned. My siblings tried to drag me into their melodramas, but because of all the work I had done on myself, neither of them could. Years ago, I would have cried and wondered how they could be so cruel, but now I felt sorry for both of them.

Sitting alone beside my mother, I thought how her womb had been my first home, just like my siblings before me, and yet I was so different from the three of them. *Did my siblings have the ability to see who among us has been acting the most mature and loving?*

They both chose to trust this facility, which was their right to do. I couldn't and wouldn't, which was my right as well. The problem was that they kept insisting that I act and think like them. They didn't realize how ridiculous it was to expect this of anyone. They had been using this same controlling tactic ever since I got sick. It didn't work before, and it's not working now. And yet they couldn't see this mistake that they kept making for years?

Before I got radiation damage, I found my mother staring out her kitchen window in a daze. Her husband was bedridden, dying of lung cancer, unable to breathe. Frantically, he was calling for her help. I just happened to walk in the front door to visit them when I heard him screaming. I dialed 911 and quickly, a policeman arrived with oxygen. My mother had become paralyzed from hearing her husband's screams, much like her own screams seemed to have paralyzed my two siblings as Mom was dying. So all three of them got overwhelmed easily, and this is why they couldn't think rationally?

Most people don't realize that someone doesn't have to be an addict for her life to be turned upside down by addictions. I'm not an addict or an alcoholic, and I don't think either of my siblings are. But we learned many of the same unhealthy habits that have affected our lives since childhood. This is why there are meetings for adult children of alcoholics, and not just meetings for alcoholics.

Because of our parents' inability to address their children's emotional needs, my siblings and I grew up living in pain and confusion. I was three years old when I opened the door of our refrigerator and a large glass bottle of milk fell and smashed by my feet. Terrified, I burst into tears.

Rather than comforting their frightened young child, my father grabbed a camera and took a photograph while my mother laughed. I stood watching in confusion, shaking in fear. This photo, glued into our family album is labeled, "No use crying over spilled milk," and it still makes me shudder each time I see it.

Had my siblings learned from my parents to detach themselves in a similar way? My mother's torturous death and the way my family treated me after I got radiation damage created more pain and agony than all my health problems combined. Emotionally, I was gutted. But keeping my heart open and being determined to understand what made them act the way they did kept me from growing angry and bitter.

No one should ever have to die in pain the way my mother did, or have to watch anyone die like this, let alone their own mother screaming in agony for days. Seeing the pleading in my mother's eyes and hearing her screams day after day and not being able to help her is something I'll always remember and and will have to live with for the rest of my life.

Addictions are currently affecting billions of innocent people all over the world, creating divisions within families, just like mine. By showing how addictions affected me and my family after I got sick, I hope to bring awareness to this growing problem and to eradicate or at least help to decrease the pain and suffering that many people experience.

While sitting alone by my mother's bedside, I realized that my siblings were acting the way our mother taught them to act. They were simply mimicking her.

During the week of my mother's passing, I had to accept that no matter how much love I shared, how much I supported my siblings, and how much respect I showed them, it would never be enough, because I couldn't stop their pain and anger. No one could convince them that their reality was distorted until they were willing to consider this.

We were all created with free will, which gives us the ability to think for ourselves. In the documentary, *I Am Not Your Negro*, James Baldwin explains why so much anger exists. He said, "Not everything that is faced can be changed, but nothing can be changed until it is faced."

It takes a lot of courage to look at yourself and take responsibility for the choices you make so you can grow into the adult you want to be. Being born with free will gives us all the choice of awakening ... or not. How we decide to live our lives is up to each of us. Some of us strive for unity, peace, and unconditional love, and some of us simply don't.

Isn't it ironic that when we look at our unflattering and most vulnerable sides, we expand our self-awareness and appreciation for ourselves? And we gain more confidence, happiness, and our lives become filled with more love.

Be Your Authentic Self

When we sacrifice who we are to please others, we weaken ourselves and our bodies. You can't afford to do this. During my healing journey, others were always trying to change me in what seemed like a desperate attempt to find the security they themselves needed. Regardless of what others may want, always strive to be yourself.

Make a list of the ways you maintained who you are without giving yourself away to please others. How did this feel when you maintained your dignity? Could you feel your body strengthen and your confidence improve?

_____

_____

_____

_____

_____

_____

_____

In what ways did you give in to what someone else wanted? Why were you unable to be true to yourself? What made others' needs more important? And how do you wish you could have acted and will do better in the future?

_____

_____

_____

_____

_____

_____

_____

_____

34

Creating the Love You Want and Need

Before I left for Florida, I heard an impressive poet named Margaret Gibson read poems from her book *Broken Cup* that she had written about her husband's slow decline from Alzheimer's. She masterfully described the pain of her heart breaking. She ended one poem by saying, "But the good thing about this is it made me tender."

Pain shot through my body when I heard these words. Warm tears streamed down my cheeks as I tried to hide my face using my hands and hair. As I was sitting among her large admiring audience, I was annoyed that the lighting was so bright, and that people could see me—as I wished my family had grown tender, too, for both their sake and mine.

***

After hospice arrived, I heard my brother and his wife making plans to leave. Since my sister had made it clear that she preferred having Mom to herself, as hard as this was, I decided the most loving thing I could do for her, and the most responsible thing I could do for my weakened body, was to go home and get the rest I needed.

Being over a thousand miles from my dying mother while recuperating from this emotional week was much harder than I thought it would be. In my mind's eye, I kept seeing my sister in her fragile state as she clung to both our mother's hands.

In an attempt to make this easier for her, I emailed hospice's social worker and asked if she would assure my sister that the facility had done nothing wrong, maybe even tell her that I had only been an Expressive Arts Specialist for hospice and didn't know as much as I thought I did.

In less than an hour, my sister sent me an email that simply read, "There was nothing wrong with the facility!"

Rather than feeling relieved and gaining strength from this, she chose to lash out at me in anger. At least my sister no longer had to wonder about the competence of that god-awful place. I had relieved her of this. Since this had to make her feel better and this was my intention, I still felt victorious.

Days later, I received another email from her telling me that Mom had died. What a cold and painful way to learn of my mother's passing.

"Sandi, you really don't regret making the sacrifice you made to help clear your sister's guilt?" a friend asked.

"Our mother used guilt to discipline us when we were growing up, so all three of us still suffer from it. It's something I've fought all my life. But my sister suffers even more from this because she now uses guilt like our mother did in an attempt to control others."

"But this was still a pretty big sacrifice you made for your sister."

"She thought she could make the decisions about our mother's passing on her own. But she couldn't, and she'll always suffer for this. I wanted to do something to help her. I'd rather decrease her guilt and have her be angry with me. After all, being angry with me is nothing new."

"In what way did your sister support you while your mother was dying?"

"She let me stay in her home while I was there," I answered, eager to say something positive.

"But like your mother, it seems to me that your sister has a difficult time giving of herself. And feeling grateful for anything you do. She sounds emotionally blocked, like my sister who's an alcoholic and blames everyone for her problems."

***

As a little girl, filled with hope and enthusiasm, I viewed the world as if it were an exhilarating scavenger hunt with millions of treasures just waiting to be found. Knowing there was a God watching over me gave me the confidence to push myself in search of what I knew I was meant to discover.

It felt wonderful to have the ability to make my mother laugh when I was young, and bring these moments of lightness and happiness into our home. Feeling special in her eyes helped me to prepare myself for the challenges ahead. My poor health terrified my mother, and she resented me for this. She never understood that she was terrified because she didn't know how to cope with her emotions, not because of anything that I did to her.

"You don't love me," she accused me not long before she died.

"I love you, Mom, as much as I love anyone in the world, probably more, but I don't like the way you've treated me since I got radiation damage. Perhaps this is what's confusing you," I said, and waited for her to reply. But there was only silence.

Because my mother was who she was, I have become a better person. I now know how deeply I can love someone, the depth of my patience, and my willingness to keep my mind and heart open and attempt to understand others. Since I grew up feeling deserted by my father, I used to fear I would be like him. Discovering these traits I have, the depth of my love and my loyalty, has been especially significant to me.

It was because I loved my family that I had become so driven to understand them. It was my love for each of them that made me determined to know what had cast such a dark and ominous shadow that blocked their hearts. I had to know what caused them to turn against me after I got sick. I knew they had loved me before I got radiation damage. I had never once questioned their love before. Because the members of my family so drastically changed and wouldn't tell me why, part of my healing journey was to understand and make peace with the choices they made as best I could.

The more I learned about addictions and how they affected whole families, I pledged to never get caught in the same traps that ensnared the three of them, filling their lives with bitterness and nonstop anger.

It was because I had to understand how it was possible for their thinking to become so distorted, that my understanding of people, the world, and my place in it exponentially expanded. As painful as it was to feel my mother's heart grow cold, the love I felt from her—before I got radiation damage—will always be a part of the person I am. Even after experiencing the agonizing void her drug use created—and the changes in my siblings—I never questioned my love for them. I'll never stop loving my family, regardless of how they feel about me. I really don't think they chose to be such angry, unhappy people.

It was from Eckhart Tolle that I learned this: "It is misleading to say that somebody 'chose' a dysfunctional relationship or any other negative situation in his or her life. Choice implies consciousness, a high degree of consciousness. Without it, you have no choice. Choice begins the moment you dis-identify from the mind and its conditioned patterns, the moment you become present. Until you reach that point, you are unconscious, spiritually speaking. This means that you are compelled to think, feel, and act in certain ways, according to the conditioning of your mind. That is why Jesus said: 'Forgive them, for they know not what they do.' "

My mother's dying gave me an invaluable opportunity to see that I could cope with my grief with strength, dignity, and maturity. It gave me an opportunity to see how much I learned from the pain I endured.

To be able to live after a death sentence was placed on me, I had to teach myself to follow my heart no matter what. I was able to support my mother as she was dying, support my siblings, and take care of myself because love opened doors. I simply walked through them.

My only goal was to share my love. If I were an only child, I would have never seen how much I had grown or understood why choosing love to guide me would upset anyone. Because I have siblings, I now understand: since love has become the focus of my life, I have obtained what neither of them have. I wish they had the ability to take responsibility for themselves and never have the need to blame anyone, so they could have grown and flourished with me.

Author Brené Brown said, "Blame is simply the discharging of discomfort and pain." And sadly, this is what my siblings repeatedly do, having learned this from our mother. So they remain stuck and do not grow.

All the work I did after I got sick got validated in a way that only my siblings could have confirmed for me. They may be far from perfect, but they've been perfect for helping me see that the goal I made in 1987—to let love guide me—helped me in more ways than I ever dreamed of. I saturated every cell in my body with love to give me strength to assist my mother on the journey she was about to take. And I used love to help my siblings, too, to protect and strengthen them as best I could.

Two days after I returned home, I had dinner with a friend who worked for hospice as a social worker for over 30 years. When Sharon saw how exhausted I looked, she gave me a loving pep talk.

"Often people put off calling hospice because it means that death is near. They justify their actions which, of course, isn't good for the dying person."

I really do understand this and don't blame my sister.

"What was obvious to you, your siblings couldn't see. Only you knew how much easier hospice would have made everything. Fighting like you did to help your mother was something no one should ever have to do, but you'll always remember what you did for her."

"It was so sad that they didn't know any better and they thought they knew all they needed to know," I said. "Then again, this is their pattern."

"But your siblings had to notice, or at least in hindsight, that they were the ones yelling at such an inappropriate time. They'll probably realize and call you and apologize this week, don't you think?"

"This would require that they take responsibility for their behavior. I don't think they're capable of doing this. They haven't yet anyway, after all these years."

After my mother died, I wondered if the facility learned anything from my exposing their deficiencies because I had screamed for days about the insufficient care my mother was receiving. I was curious to know if anyone there had ever reviewed their actions. I read on their website that "30-day rehabilitation from substance abuse" was no longer offered. Never again will anyone have to experience what my mother, my two siblings, and I did.

I cried.

When You Open Your Heart and Witness, Your Whole Life Changes

After I learned how to regulate my nervous system, it was much easier to remember to live with an open heart. Regulating myself helped me to ground myself and witness reality, as well as make better decisions. Learn to regulate your nervous system and avoid engaging with people who are emotionally dysregulated.

If you haven't already, teach yourself to regulate your nervous system. Make a list of the benefits to this.

_____

_____

_____

_____

_____

_____

_____

This is a process. There will still be many times you'll forget and resort to your old habits. List each time you weren't successful, ways that will help you do better in the future, and what not being regulated has cost you.

_____

_____

_____

_____

_____

_____

_____

35

Needs Are Needs

"You do agree it should just be the three of us? And where do you think we ought to spread Mom's ashes?" my sister emailed me five months after our mother's death, and a month before the weekend of her service.

My sister had emailed me previously that we were scattering the ashes by boat, so I was confused by her question. I was delighted that my opinion was at last being asked, and that I was being recognized as Mom's daughter too who deserved to have some say-so.

The week our mother was dying, my sister announced she wanted to oversee Mom's memorial service. To my surprise, she said she had already started writing the eulogy. I told her I had no objection, but she also took control of spreading Mom's ashes without further discussion.

When she wrote and asked for my opinion, I read this as a good sign that she was healing because her world was expanding beyond herself.

"Yes, I do agree it should just be the three of us. I think East Dock would be a good place to spread Mom's ashes," I emailed back.

As if the Hoover dam had broken, thoughts about this day flooded my mind. Because of the damage to my neurological system, my body could still become sensitive and out-of-balance if I didn't take extra care of myself. This often required that I plan ahead to avoid problems.

Because it took me so long to recover after I returned from Florida, I was grateful for my sister's email reminding me to start preparing for this weekend now. This would be a day I would always remember, and the last thing I wanted was my health to interfere.

I pictured the three of us silently walking to East Dock, the same dock I fished from when I was young, where I had once imagined my own funeral would be. It was clear I wouldn't get any more writing done, so I allowed my thoughts to wander. Just because my mother got addicted to drugs, it wasn't her fault that she trusted her doctor when he told her opioids were not addictive.

An estimated two million people got addicted during the opioid crisis. With all the aches, pains, and physical problems Mom had, and being so emotionally challenged, I could now understand how this happened.

I also realized there was more to my mother's life beyond me, and she deserved to be honored as the person God created and loved. She never appreciated this about herself, which was why I focused on this. I wanted to celebrate her and the many contributions she had made to my life. My hope was to say something that explained this during this last precious chance I got to honor her. I began composing what I would say before we spread her ashes. I felt a belonging-to-a-family kind of feeling; one I hadn't expected to feel this day. As my eyes got teary, I sat in silence and enjoyed this.

All that was left of our family was just my two siblings and me. I pictured the three of us together, being reverential, not just for our mother, but out of respect for one another, and in a larger sense, as a way of honoring the sanctity of families throughout the world. We would be partaking in a ritual that every person, since the beginning of mankind, has or will participate in, in one form or another. All throughout history, families have been honoring the passing of their loved ones. Now it was our turn to become part of this historic, solemn, and influential occasion.

In the following months, had my siblings recognized that I had also been grieving for our mother while we were together in Florida? Had they realized that they used me—during this vulnerable time—just because they had to vent? Or had they found some way to justify their behavior, just as they had always done?

I wanted to believe it was possible that they could now see how awful they'd treated me. And they would want to make up for this by being extra kind when we got together. I looked forward to seeing them and being a part of my family again. I hoped that I would be respected and treated as a contributing one third.

I chuckled at the irony of my mother's death bringing us closer after she kept us separated and fighting all her life. She was never comfortable having two of us in the same room with her, giving each other the attention that she craved.

"I think she's afraid we'll gang up on her. I can't imagine being so insecure you fear your own children and make sure they don't like each other for your own benefit," my sister had told me when she was 21 years old and had decided to put an end to this.

I was a freshman at Boston University. She was a senior at Northeastern. I was elated when she invited me for dinner in her very first apartment and she told me that we ought to be friends. But this didn't last long. Maybe now, with our mother gone, she'd make another effort to overcome how Mom had programmed her.

I pictured the three of us standing side-by-side on the long wooden dock after we each said what we wanted to say to mark the end of our mother's life. On the count of three, I envisioned the three of us tipping the urn as Mom's ashes fell into the blue salt water, leaving a long line of light gray ash that bobbed up and down with the small choppy waves.

I saw us standing in silence, watching as the ashes floated farther and farther away from us. The only sound that could be heard was a lone seagull crying. Out of respect, each of us would give one another a moment to stop and remember this complex, unique, tortured, intelligent, creative, and beautiful woman.

Only we knew the harrowing challenges she'd wrestled with. How much she'd suffered because she'd never learned to love herself. She never could let go of a deep-rooted core belief that she wasn't good enough. And yet she'd yearned to be. She'd wanted so badly to feel loved. No matter how hard I tried, I could never convince her how much she was truly loved.

Ever since her death, I had been focusing on the sweet times we shared prior to her addiction, when I was young and she lit up my life. I thought about how much we enjoyed singing harmony in church, and how we appreciated each other's sense of humor. As painful as this was, I had spent these past five months since her death focusing on how much I loved her. And how hard I had tried to bring us closer again. Despite how many tears these thoughts created, it left me feeling grateful for my mother and for everything she had done for me.

Prompted by my sister's unexpected email, I wondered how my brother was coping. I hoped, for his sake, that he wasn't emotionally grappling. And I hoped that he'd found strength within himself to face and feel his pain—that it wasn't overwhelming and devouring the poor guy. I hoped he wouldn't have to use his sense of humor to distract himself from feeling his feelings, like he usually did.

I wondered if it was possible for him to keep this ritual sacred, out of respect for Mom and the rest of us who were grieving. With his emotions eating away at him, was he even capable of considering that his two sisters had lost their mother, too? Since my sister knew raising children required sacrifice, I was sure she would set a respectful example.

Still sitting in front of my computer, I was thinking about the three of us getting together to honor the first person in our family from our original four-person unit that we had lost. Who would die next? Would my siblings even care if it was me? Would they regret how cruelly they had treated me?

Since having control gave my sister security, I was not about to interfere with whatever she planned. Whenever she went into control mode, I had learned long ago to keep a safe distance. Nonetheless, I was surprised when I received an email from her months before telling me the date of Mom's funeral. Since the date worked for her, was this all she thought about?

As this weekend approached, she kept emailing me contradictory information. To keep my body from getting stressed, I had to have a better idea as to what to expect, so I emailed her and requested, as politely as I could, that if any changes were made, to please keep me updated.

The next email I received from her was on the morning of this long-awaited day, telling me that my car was needed since everyone couldn't fit into her rental. I was given instructions to meet at the Taber Inn in Mystic. From here we would take two cars to a designated spot in Groton Long Point where my brother and his wife, my sister and her husband, their two sons, one's wife and one's fiancé (whom I had never met), and I proceeded to walk to East Dock.

Remember to keep your heart open. Feel the love that's always there.

As we walked together, I was silently rehearsing what I would say when it was my turn to speak. I was nervous and hoped that I didn't flub it up. *Just speak from your heart*, I kept telling myself.

At the intersection of Crescent Street and South Shore Road, those ahead of me turned right, not in the direction of East Dock. *Where the heck were we going?* I was annoyed but quickly told myself the healthiest thing I could do was not to resist whatever happened on this day. Go with the flow and ride with the tide.

When we reached the far end of South Beach, my brother-in-law and brother broke from the group. Merrily they skipped along the water's edge while twirling, giggling, and swinging their arms over their heads, throwing handfuls of Mom's ashes high in the air.

To stop myself from crying, I took long slow breaths. As I watched in horror, I told myself: *Everyone has the right to honor Mom however they choose.* The dancing seemed to go on and on as I stood watching while trying to keep my heart open.

But this isn't even where Mom liked to sit. She never sat at this end of the beach where the crowds were. She preferred her privacy at the opposite end, I thought as I studied the two dancing men more closely and silently apologized to my mother for leaving her where she would not be comfortable.

Their movements were stiff and awkward. Their sappy smiles looked strained and fake, signs that both of them were having trouble coping with their grief.

They were using humor to create a smokescreen to hide behind. Rather than learning to cope with their emotions, this is the strategy they used to compensate. And they thought no one would notice?

I felt sorry for them. My disgust turned to compassion. It was so sad that these two grown men lived their lives so handicapped. They both had so many admirable talents and good traits but they both suffered emotionally.

As if she wanted to quickly get it over with, seconds after we walked onto East Dock, my sister, struggling to compose herself, read a passage from the Bible. Standing just a few feet from her, I was sincerely trying to understand how this reading related to our mother. As I stood waiting for my sister to ask who wanted to speak next, I was startled by yet another surprise. *My sister was shouting!*

She was scolding her husband in an abrasive voice. In return, he was quick to reply, "You don't want me here? Fine. I'll just move if this will make you happy, dear," while he was displaying the same sappy fake grin as before, trying to look calm and in control, although his expression loudly announced that he wasn't.

Just minutes ago, his wife was crying over the death of her mother. And he wasn't being protective of her? Partners are supposed to be supportive of each other, especially at times like this. But didn't he know to put his grieving wife first?

And how could the two of them be so oblivious? How is it possible that they'd forgotten that there were other people here who were also grieving? Or was the problem that they just didn't care?

Keep your heart open and connect with this love.

My brother-in-law must have become overwhelmed by his feelings, so he took his discomfort out on my sister. This is how my siblings usually treat me. My brother, sister, and my brother-in-law all acted so immaturely. It was painful to watch.

Pieces were falling together: My sister did not have a partner who could emotionally support her. How could she not feel unseen and abandoned? And no doubt, this wasn't the first time—which would explain why she'd grown more resentful and bitter the older she'd become. And also why she was so desperate to get what she wanted.

Because my poor sister had not been receiving emotional support at quintessential times like this, it explained why she hadn't supported me when I got sick. She'd treated me the way that she'd been treated by both our parents ... and by her husband, too. She probably thought I should have grown a thick skin, just like she had. But this creates bitterness.

I was still patiently waiting for her to ask who wanted to speak next when over to my right I heard a loud splash. *Oh no! Someone fell in the water?!* I used to teach junior lifesaving, so by habit I was about to take off my shoes, just in case I needed to jump in the water to help. Then I realized what caused this splash. My brother-in-law had thrown my mother's urn into the water!

My mind exploded. Frantically, I searched for ways to make sense of what had just happened: Had he done this in anger, to show my sister he was the one in control? Or had my sister changed plans again without telling me? Had she decided to give her husband this honor without asking me if this was alright? I could see her doing this, but would my brother-in-law intrude like this, just assume he had the right?

I felt weak. My balance was wobbly. I clung onto the nearest wooden piling to keep myself from falling. I kept my eyes glued on my mother's urn and watched as it was quickly pulled out to sea by the current, growing smaller and smaller, as more distance between us grew. I was still in shock, but I kept my focus on my mother's urn for as long as I could. Only when I could no longer see the tiny speck it had become did I let go of the piling.

Bewildered. Disoriented. Dazed. I turned and widened my stance to steady myself. Walking like a duck to balance myself and keep myself from falling, I made my way back slowly and carefully onto the safety of dry land.

I saw my sister passing on my left. Too stunned to properly form my thoughts, I asked her why he'd done that.

"Who? Did what?" she asked as she slowed her pace.

"Why did he throw Mom's urn in the water?

"What? You weren't upset by that, were you?"

"He had his own mother's funeral after she died. Why would he impose himself into ours? You told me the three of us were going to do this."

My sister turned and scurried away.

Be Present

When my thoughts are judgmental, I can feel my body reacting like a pinball machine blaring "tilt," signaling it's time to rebalance and be present ... and open my heart. After feeling disgust for the two frolicking men throwing my mother's ashes, I told myself that everyone had a right to honor my mother however they chose, and my body relaxed. By realigning myself in this way, expanding my thinking and my heart, I became present to what gave me a far more accurate understanding of what was really happening.

When you pay attention to how your body feels, it will tell you when you're going in the wrong direction. The longer you commit yourself to following love, the more your body will help you stay on this path. List each time your body helps you go in a healthier direction.

_____

_____

_____

_____

_____

_____

_____

List the times you didn't listen, and you brought discomfort into your life. Why and what did this cost you? What will you do differently next time?

_____

_____

_____

_____

_____

_____

36

Looking Through the Lens of Love, You'll See and Gain So Much More

The memorial service was the next day. I awoke feeling weak and nauseous. I knew if I went, I'd be pushing myself, but out of respect for my mother and siblings, I got dressed and drove to the church.

My mother had been a popular schoolteacher for almost 20 years. She taught in two elementary schools just minutes from where her service was about to be held. I had thought we should invite the public, but my sister had insisted on family only.

"Then why have it in Connecticut? Why not in Florida?" I asked her more than once, but my question was never answered. I could only guess, knowing how my sister thought, that she wanted to vacation in New England with her husband and two boys so they could enjoy the beautiful fall foliage and eat McIntosh apples from Clyde's Cider Mill, apples that my sister loved.

As I entered St. Mark's Episcopal Church, my body trembled when I saw the cold and desolate emptiness, the nearly vacant brown wooden pews. Seeing the church looking this sad and pathetic, I had to hold back my tears.

Remember to keep your heart open. Feel the love.

There were no colorful flowers on the altar or anywhere to give the church life. My mother used to be on this church's flower guild. Why were there no flowers for her today? Only a few clusters of people were scattered about.

A sickening hollow emptiness crept over my body. I was forced to feel the depth of bitterness in my sister's heart. As I walked down the center aisle and took my seat in the front row beside her, I felt sick. I had wanted this church filled with people from the many parts of my mother's long life. I wanted them here to remember this woman who taught me how deeply I could love.

"She's not a real Christian. She studies the Bible and knows it well, but she doesn't know its true meaning," my sister told me the week Mom was dying. And yet she believed this service represented the true meaning of Christ?

This empty church represented her own strained relationship she had with Mom. Despite having a brother and sister whose mother was also being remembered today, what my sister had planned was all about her.

Horses are often forced to wear blinders to keep their eyes focused forward. The way our brains are designed for our survival, when humans become stressed, we become myopic. This is usually just temporary. The stress my sister lived with not only caused her to become shortsighted, but it was clear that her stress affected how she both thought and lived her life. On this day that was supposed to be about my mother, my sister's anger was screaming in my face.

A loved one's addiction can be horrible and brutal. It affects our lives in many negative ways, but I still expected my sister to look beyond herself and consider all the years that Mom had lived. *Please don't let my sister be in as much pain as I'm seeing. This is really breaking my heart. I don't know how much more I can take.*

I don't believe life happens to us, but for us. If we view our challenges as lessons, they help us develop in the ways we need. If we choose to learn from them, and not get stuck in our anger or steep ourselves in self-pity, everything we experience can be beneficial. My sister had gotten stuck and so she suffered. And she refused to change for some reason. It was as if she felt she didn't deserve to be happy. She was so much like our mother in this way.

So, what am I to learn from this gruesome experience? Maybe this weekend has been as painful as it's been, to remind me of how narrow my perspective becomes if I don't keep my heart open. Please Lord, give me strength to keep my heart open.

As much as I tried, I couldn't ignore the weird and twisted pleasure that was emanating from my sister, who was grinning as she sat next to me.

I think it was because of her grin that I remembered, while sitting there, that my sister's sixth grade teacher had chosen her to play the evil queen in Snow White, who asked the mirror who was the fairest of them all. My brother and I had both laughed at this because we thought the role was perfect for her. But while I was sitting in the church, I no longer thought it was funny because it proved to be a harbinger of this very moment.

She had always been insecure and jealous since she was young, but now this had grown as if it was on steroids.

Since I lived just minutes from where I grew up, people often told me how much they loved having my mother as their teacher. This is why I wanted the church to be filled with her students' love and appreciation.

"Everywhere I've taken Mom, people have loved her: her doctors, everyone at the rehabilitation center, the assisted living facility. She did superficial relationships well. She just couldn't handle intimacy," my sister told me years before, looking like a sad little girl who had never gotten the love she wanted from her mommy.

I had forgiven my mother long ago for how she had treated me; otherwise, like a piece of bacon in a frying pan, I too might be sizzling in anger. Never would I have been able to improve my health and obtained so much happiness.

At the designated time, my sister rose from the pew and stood behind the podium, grinning in an overly exaggerated manner, as she faced the tiny congregation. Clasping both hands tightly on the podium, she leaned her body forward as if to do a pushup. Slowly, she glided her body from left to right as she swept her eyes across the audience in a theatrical way.

Like a small child excited to have everyone's attention, and about to burst from some revelation she'd been waiting to share for years, my sister said, "You may remember my mother as a schoolteacher or perhaps an aunt or whatever, but she also had a side to her that many of you don't know."

While still grinning in a determined manner that I found uncomfortable to watch, she told unflattering stories about our mother, such as how Mom used to cover her windows with dark paper at night so no one knew she was home. And the time our mother missed her exit on the I-95, but she exited anyway by driving up the steep embankment while we, her frightened passengers, prayed for our lives.

My sister had nothing kind to say about our mother. Couldn't she have said something like:

My mother was always generous to me.

I'll always be grateful to her for being the best babysitter I ever had when I was a young mother, struggling and needing a break from my two boys.

I'm so very appreciative of both the time and all the things she gave my boys—she even took my youngest son on a trip to Hawaii once. My mother gave them both things they would have otherwise gone without.

She was a wonderful cook and made my family many great meals.

When my sister finished telling unkind stories about our mother, she held her chin high, looking proud of herself for what she'd accomplished. She had been planning for over a year to stab Mom in the back? Could she not speak her truth to anyone and gotten some guidance? I felt hot and dizzy.

Before my sister had even seated herself, my sister-in-law jumped up from her pew. Though English wasn't her first language and she often stumbled as she searched for words, the heartfelt way she expressed her love for my mother was refreshing and endearing, especially since there was a time my mother had forbidden her to come to Groton Long Point because "people pay taxes to keep people like her out."

I so wished that I too, could have spoken, but my body was screaming to be cared for. It had been pushed way too far. Once the service was over, like Cinderella having to leave before the clock struck 12, I had to make a quick exit. Before leaving, I told my sister I had to go while I could still drive.

"Are you alright?" she asked, to which I answered with an honest no. And yet this is the last conversation I ever had with my sister.

Just a few blocks from the church, a policeman pulled me over for stopping at a green light. (The brain tumor had given me dyslexic symptoms that surfaced whenever I was stressed, so the green light registered in my brain as red.) Yelling that he had almost rear-ended me as he approached my car window, he couldn't have been kinder after I told him I had just come from my mother's memorial service.

Despite my best efforts to prepare myself for this weekend, my body rebelled for months: multiple doctors' visits, batteries of tests, trips to the hospital, and extensive medical bills followed. My health became central to my life again.

When a biopsy of my thyroid came back questionable, because it was so close to where radiation had damaged my brain, my doctor wanted to operate, but I declined. Arterial-venous malformations (AVM) were found scattered throughout my intestines and had been bleeding for who knows how long. Each one had to be cauterized because the bleeding had caused severe anemia, which exacerbated the chronic fatigue syndrome, and a cacophony of other problems, which I won't bore my readers by listing.

221

We reap the most rewards when we allow life to unfold without insisting like a child that life goes our way. I have found that one of the best ways to help my body heal was by accepting each situation to be what it was instead of what I wanted—as difficult as this could be at times. Once I was accepting, I could relax, and because thinking was much easier, I made better decisions. "Accepting" is the key word here.

I kept resisting seeing the depth of my sister's misery because it felt so painful. This caused stress on my body and I knew I would suffer the consequences. Much like my sister expecting more than our mother could give, I had been expecting more than she was capable of. All weekend long, I had been forced to see how deeply my sister suffered, but I stubbornly resisted this because I love her.

I had learned my lesson: I had to let go and accept her choice to live her life in whatever way she chose. I still shudder to think that for years I believed that because of the brutal way my family treated me, I wasn't worthy of their love. That something had to be wrong with me. Because my family acted like they wished I had died, there were times I thought that perhaps I should have.

Forgiving myself for the pain my illness caused my family has not been easy. They were responsible for how they reacted, but there was no denying that my getting sick was difficult on them. Whether it was due to their emotional deficiencies or not, each of them suffered, and I wish they hadn't.

When I have told my friends how badly I felt, every one of them said the same thing: that my family hurt me more than I could have possibly hurt them. Even if this is true, pain is pain and my family experienced pain after I got sick.

It's true they made no effort to help themselves. They could have gotten professional help, but because they didn't, this was a major contributor to their suffering. And none of them ever stopped playing the victim, and they encouraged each other to do it, which only made their problems worse. But refusing to take responsibility for their behavior is what contributed to their pain the most, and sadly, it continues to.

I love my family and I'm sorry they never learned their self-worth and realized they deserved more than they allowed themselves to have. It pained me to watch them act like they didn't deserve happiness. If I hadn't spent years trying to understand them and forgiven myself for the pain they felt, I would never have healed as fully as I have. Forgiving myself for hurting them, whether others think it was appropriate or not, was a crucial part of my healing process. This was something I had to do for myself, not for my family.

I'm sure this won't surprise anyone, but I also grew up with emotional deficiencies. After all, I lived in the same home that my two siblings did. No one magically escapes being affected by the dysfunctions in their homes. Some people hide this better than others using humor, for example, or having a job helping others so they feel and appear altruistic. But unless their dysfunctional behavior is addressed, their pain and frustration will only increase. This is our body's way of telling us it needs our attention.

"As long as you keep secrets and suppress information, you are fundamentally at war with yourself ... The critical issue is allowing yourself to know what you know. That takes an enormous amount of courage," wrote Bessel van der Kolk in *The Body Keeps the Score: Brain, Mind, and Body in the Healing of Trauma*.

None of my mother's three children got their emotional needs met in childhood. And each of us has suffered because of this. It took a double whammy—living with Gary and getting the brain tumor—for me to realize I needed to take a good look at myself and make the needed changes.

Initially, I began attending 12-step meetings in 1989 because I wanted to learn how to make my relationship with Gary work. But at the very first meeting I attended, I realized I had a lot of work to do on myself. I still remember hearing that in most relationships where addictions were involved, caring for an addicted partner provided us with a sense of purpose and that we often derived our identity from this self-sacrifice. My body cringed when I heard this, signaling me to pay strict attention.

My mother expected her three children to spend their lives sacrificing for her, which is yet another reason why my family became so angry with me: After I got sick, I could no longer afford to make these life-draining sacrifices, or I would have never gotten well. Lori had taught me how unhealthy this was. Once I understood what this was costing me, it became clear I had to break this lifelong habit.

No one else in my family had ever learned it was unhealthy and irresponsible to sacrifice more than we could afford to lose. Sacrificing was how the members of my family derived their identity and expressed their love. It was how they saw themselves as good people. Because I was no longer acting how my family believed good people act, they punished me.

Thankfully, at the first 12-step meeting I attended, I was willing to consider that I could be contributing to my problems, and to not just view Gary as the problem. Being willing to look at our behavior is a crucial step for us to heal.

It wasn't until 2017, when I was surprised that my brother-in-law didn't know to support his wife as she was grieving her mother's death, that I realized how far-reaching the tentacles of addictions had enhanced my sister's and my entire family's problems. Addictions ran in my sister's husband's family, too, and he had unresolved deficiencies as well. For over 30 years, my sister had been suffering from the effects of addictions from both her husband's family and her own. And she had never gotten help for herself.

Since the two of them lacked emotional maturity because they never learned how to cope with their emotions in an effective way, they both became challenged on the dock. Since my sister hadn't gotten her fundamental needs met as a child or as an adult, she had been suffering all her life. It became clear she had been sacrificing parts of herself (just like I used to do), trying to make her marriage work. When I saw this, bells and whistles went off in my head.

Before I stood on East Dock to honor my mother, I thought I understood the problems my family had, but I had only seen the tip of the iceberg. That sickening, stomach-turning moment when I heard the splash of my mother's urn striking the water affirmed what I had fought for decades not to see—the extent of my family's pain and dysfunction. And the good job they had done covering this up.

When I could no longer avoid seeing this, and was capable of feeling this pain, I was standing on the same dock surrounded by the same supportive and expansive sea that had nurtured me since I was young. This was the same fortifying vastness from the same blue sky overhead where I had spent hours as a child embraced by Mother Nature.

When I gathered with my family, believing that I was about to participate in the sacred ritual of spreading my mother's ashes, I was standing on the same dock where I was also given strength, peace, and love as a middle-aged woman battling the frightening symptoms from radiation damage.

During this intense volcanic moment the splashing of the urn created, I don't think it was a coincidence that I was supported by the same familiar environment once again. Because I kept my heart open, didn't get angry or feel sorry for myself, and did my best to accept the way my family acted, I was able to comprehend what was happening while it was unfurling before me.

As my mother's ashes were carried out to sea, like a phoenix rising, I experienced a rebirth. Thanks to my sister and brother-in-law and the challenges they faced, I was given vivid clarity: to expect anything more from my family was futile. Supporting each other on this day, when most people knew to care for one another and to treat each other with maximum kindness, was foreign to my family. This was the world they lived in. But it was foreign to me.

What I had been striving for years to understand was acted out in front of me as if I watching a Broadway show, as if they were on stage and I was sitting in the audience. I observed how they shielded themselves from each other's needs in the same way they had protected themselves from my needs when my health threatened them.

Like Gary, my family's inclination was to not resolve problems. Instead, they blamed others for the problems they had.

At last, I realized that my family couldn't have possibly helped me after I got sick because they didn't know how to help themselves.

Why Choose Love to Guide You?

Love heals. Your immune system strengthens when you feel love. Love helps stabilize your mood and allows you to trust, accept, and forgive. Love inspires you to improve your behavior, break your bad habits and get help for yourself, leading you down a path of self-discovery. Love encourages your creativity. It helps you think outside of the box and find creative solutions to problems. Love increases happiness, reduces anxiety, and makes you feel safe and secure. And love connects you to yourself and others, adding more love to your life.

Notice how often you feel love. Where in your body do you feel this and in what ways and when?

_____

_____

_____

_____

_____

_____

_____

Why might you find it challenging at times to feel love? What might you do to increase the ability of love to flow into your body and life? What ways might you remind yourself to keep your heart open?

_____

_____

_____

_____

_____

_____

_____

37

Find What Works for You

My life has been filled with happiness and sorrow, fear and pain, and more love than I ever imagined was possible. Every one of us is given nights and days, summers, winters, springs, and falls, and high and low tides as reminders that life changes every day, and that since we are part of nature, we are meant to change as well.

After my doctors told me I would soon die, I yearned to feel and share as much love as I could, in whatever time I had left to live. Thankfully, most people began treating me more lovingly. And as love poured into my life, the more loved I felt, the stronger I grew.

I also became more sensitive to anything that didn't feel like love. Whenever I felt this uncomfortable lower frequency, I could feel my body contract in fear and my fears block love from flowing. I taught myself that it was to my advantage to keep my heart open. By facing, feeling, and addressing my fears—with an open heart—rather than retreating or blaming others for how I felt, I allowed myself to feel more love, and my life became less frightening. Love just naturally became an integral part of my life and has continually sculpted the woman I am.

What I hadn't realized, and was in no way prepared for, was that keeping my heart open to love would create a widening gap between my family and me. My family's priority was protecting themselves from their fears, while I was teaching myself the opposite. Their life centered around fear. Mine centered around love.

For some people, facing their fears is just too painful. They can't do it. Rather than recognizing that their fears are keeping them from experiencing the love they yearn for and the life they want, they blame others for their pain.

Some people take drugs or drink alcohol excessively, or use sex, religion, humor, food, work, shopping, anger, keeping busy, gambling, risk taking, thrill seeking, and spending money to avoid feeling pain and taking responsibility for how they feel. They don't understand that feeling their pain will free them and allow more love into their lives.

"When we see difficult circumstances as a chance to grow in bravery and wisdom, in patience and kindness, when we become more conscious of being hooked and we don't escalate it, then our personal distress can connect us with the discomfort and unhappiness of others. What we usually consider a problem becomes the source of empathy," Pema Chödrön said.

Like my siblings, I was never taught to love myself as a child. All three of us have lived with this disadvantage since we were young. After my mother's memorial service, I had to heal not just my body, but also my heart, which was grieving the loss of my mother, and how my siblings lived their lives. By having to interact with the medical world so frequently again, the PTSD I thought was behind me reared its ugly head once more.

I got jittery and felt unsafe wherever I was. I startled easily and retreated into my home, where I spent most of my time alone. I temporarily fell down the rabbit hole where old familiar feelings of unworthiness surfaced. Had I not allowed myself to feel this grief, pain, and frustration, had I not allowed myself to feel resentful that I'd been pulled back into this ugly dark place, healing from this would have taken much longer and been even more difficult.

I treated myself like the loving mother I wish I'd had, telling myself that after all the setbacks I'd had for over 20 years, this was just another bump on the road and I could handle this one, too. I told myself that feeling frustrated and resentful was a normal reaction and not to shame myself for how I felt. Just feel it and move on.

I was able to do all I had to accomplish while grieving my mother's death and my siblings' undeniable misery by strengthening myself: I incorporated self-love in my life. Every morning I wrote three things about myself that I liked. By consciously cultivating this sweet tenderness, I made loving myself a habit that became a part of my life.

This also helped me understand my siblings better. They were never taught self-love. The three of us had never been treated as if we were precious in either of our parents' eyes because our parents couldn't give us what they never got. Had I not just spent this nerve-wracking weekend with them, I would never have realized how much self-love I needed.

"Love is the most powerful force in the universe. It has the power to transform hearts, heal wounds, and create. But it all starts with loving self-love. When you love and accept unconditionally, you radiate love to others," wrote don Miguel Ruiz.

This is what led me in October 2019 to study with Scott Kiloby and learn what is called Kiloby Inquiries, and become a certified KI facilitator. I got the opportunity to work with Scott and people from all over the world to help me unearth my deepest-rooted traumas that were still interfering with my life in subtle and insidious ways. Because of this support, I no longer felt alone while facing my fears.

"Traumatic events destroy the sustaining bonds between individual and community. Those who have survived learn that their sense of self-worth, of humanity, depends upon a feeling of connection with others. The solidarity of a group provides the strongest protection against terror and despair, and the strongest antidote to traumatic experience," Judith Herman wrote in her book *Trauma and Recovery.*

This protective bond is what I experienced while practicing KI. The solidarity of this group gave me the understanding and the feeling of being connected that I had been yearning for since I'd become family-less.

Judith Herman also wrote, "Trauma isolates; the group re-creates a sense of belonging. Trauma shames and stigmatizes; the group bears witness and affirms. Trauma degrades the victim; the group exalts her. Trauma dehumanizes the victim; the group restores her humanity."

I could not be more grateful for all KI has given me. Now I understood why, for years, I thought I had to have my family's love, and why it hurt so much to be rejected. I understood why it took me so long to accept how cruelly they'd acted because after being traumatized, I yearned for this connection, protection, and sense of belonging. Now, I connected with people from all around the world on a loving and intimate level.

Practicing KI with my fellow students allowed me to safely interact with others while revealing the wounded parts of me. This was when COVID just started, so connecting to others on Zoom several times a week not only gave me back a sense of belonging, but it kept me from feeling isolated and lonely.

KI taught me how to receive answers from my body in a more specific and accessible way than I had been doing. Years of somatic (body-centered) counseling had been a huge help, but KI provided the missing key. Never before had anything offered such clarity and precision, or quickly revealed any lingering fear that was buried deep inside my body.

"Fear is a universal experience. Even the smallest insect feels it. We wade in the tidal pools and put our finger near the soft, open bodies of sea anemones and they close up," Pema Chödrön wrote in *When Things Fall Apart*.

This is exactly what I experienced whenever I felt my body contract in fear. And every time I felt my love being blocked.

Pema Chödrön continued, "Everything spontaneously does that. It's not a terrible thing that we feel fear when faced with the unknown. It is part of being alive, something we all share. We react against the possibility of loneliness, of death, of not having anything to hold on to. Fear is a natural reaction to moving closer to the truth."

The more I faced my fears and pain using KI, the more love I was able to feel. There were certain KI techniques I found particularly effective, such as the Reverse Inquiry, which got me in touch with anger I would have sworn I no longer had. By closing my eyes and saying, "I am not angry" and allowing myself to feel whatever I felt, welcoming it, offering it love and thanking it for protecting me, I could feel my body respond, perhaps with a contraction in my stomach or throat, or a sensation running across my chest.

By giving what we feel space, allowing whatever we feel, through pictures, thoughts, or feelings, our bodies speak to us. After saying, "I'm not angry," I felt a lot of energy emanating from my body. I had been doing KI for over a year, but this was the first time I got this frightened.

The amount of fear I felt with the facilitator being there for support and guidance, exposed an anger and sadness I'd been carrying. I discovered that because I had spent so many years trying to understand my family, I had overlooked the depth of my own pain and anger, and my deep sadness until this moment. The skilled facilitator working with me reminded me that feelings were just feelings and could not hurt me, which helped me to relax and allow what I felt.

"When we stop trying to make the surface calm—and accept that the very nature of [the] ocean is change—we begin to experience this inner freedom," Yongey Mingyur Rinpoche wrote in his book, *In Love with the World*. Now, whenever I feel like I'm emotionally imbalanced, I inquire into this using KI to help me access and release whatever is blocking me.

Kiloby Inquiry is not the only modality that's available to help people discover and release their fears and false beliefs and hidden traumas. I have friends (and friends of friends) who also practice Tension, Stress and Trauma Release, (TRE), Embodied Processing (EP), Somatic Experiencing (SE), Aletheia, Havening, The Judith Blackstone Realization Process, NeuroAffective Relational Model (NARM), Natural Flow Movement (NFM), to name just a few. You might want to Google Kiloby Inquiries and any of these to see if any may interest you.

No longer is my life like a fishing net, where I once became dangerously entangled, feeling like I was being held under water, not knowing if I would ever breathe again. To keep myself from drowning, I strategically found ways to free myself. Step by step, as time passed, I carefully unraveled these knotted ropes that encircled me and held my body down.

"What would you all do if you didn't have a problem? Start living and stop dying," Dr. Bernie Siegel wrote on his Facebook page, and when I read this, I cheered.

Strengthening Your Self-Awareness

Self-awareness is a necessary skill when using love to heal yourself, but you must first be curious and want to know who you are, let your walls down, and be willing to see parts of yourself that you don't like. By answering these questions at the end of each chapter, your self-awareness will increase. Meditating also helps. Ask people you trust how they see you. And whenever you have a conflict with someone, imagine yourself in the other person's shoes. By reducing your defensiveness and opening your heart, your self-awareness is sure to increase.

What are the advantages of increasing your self-awareness? How does this help you heal? Why must you be willing to see parts of yourself that you don't like?

_____

_____

_____

_____

_____

_____

What price do you pay by hiding from yourself and refusing to see your darker sides?

_____

_____

_____

_____

_____

_____

_____

A Letter to My Readers

I knew I had to write this book in much the same way I knew I had to paint the mural. I had no idea *how* I would accomplish either, only that I had to, just as I had no idea how I would save my life or overcome radiation damage or breast cancer or find peace regarding my family.

Before I painted the mural and wrote this book, I never knew how people would respond to either, nor did I give it any thought. I only focused on accomplishing both. Because I did, I learned the joys, risks, and challenges of being both a writer and an artist. I felt the compelling need both artists and writers have to express themselves. They just use different mediums.

I also discovered how easy it was to get too close to whatever I was creating. To stop ourselves from getting lost in the process of the "doing," both writers and artists must keep a distance from their work, although there are also times when getting lost and turning ourselves over to the wisdom within us is what we need to do.

Most artists start their painting using large brushstrokes, which in time become smaller and more detailed towards the end, though we don't want to get too detailed, or we'll lose the painting's overall essence, the soul of our painting. Similarly, many writers start a book with an outline and add details the more they write, being mindful not to write too much detail or not enough.

A painting hanging on a wall is typically viewed from about six feet away, which is why artists often step back from their easels and take long discerning looks at what they've painted from about this same distance. I had to be aware of my entire 63' mural while I was painting it. At times, I would climb down from my scaffolding and walk across the gallery just so I could see what I was creating.

I also had to be cognizant of my entire manuscript as I was writing. Sometimes I would set the manuscript of this book aside and come back to it later, which allowed me to understand with a fresh eye what more I needed to write and what parts were finished.

Becoming somatically sensitive (which I had to be to help save my life), gave me an unexpected advantage: Now when someone critiques my art or writing, my whole body responds in a way it never did before, giving me invaluable information. If what they say is helpful, I can feel a burst of vibrating energy inside me, as opposed to feeling a heavy thud to a suggestion that wasn't right.

Both painting and writing require the ability to express emotions. It surprised me when I discovered that this was something that came naturally to me, whether I was writing or painting. While looking at a piece of my artwork, people have often asked how I can evoke a feeling using paint. I honestly don't know, and it isn't something that's taught in school.

I have been told I can evoke feelings using words, too. I loved when my editor laughed at certain sections of this book that I'd hoped my readers would find funny. It was informative and quite satisfying to learn that certain things I wrote angered her, too.

When a reader finishes a book, one primary feeling, such as being inspired or sad, is often felt, but the feelings of the reader will change. As is evident from the people who view my paintings, a piece of art usually evokes just one prevailing feeling that most viewers feel.

I don't appreciate being force-fed under any circumstances. Therefore, whether I am painting or writing, I intentionally share my perspective and opinion, but I want my viewers and readers to form their own opinions. I think everyone's perspective is just as valid as mine. Whether I'm writing or painting, I want everyone to interpret whatever I create in their own way.

I have intentionally asked questions throughout this book, believing that we all learn and grow by thinking and considering various viewpoints, which adds depth and richness to our lives.

In both my book and mural, I told a story based on my experience, but because love, death, families, and our interactions with them are fundamental to us all, neither my book nor mural was ever meant to only be about me. I wouldn't be alive today if it weren't for other people, so this cannot be separated.

We are all a part of this world. None of us lives in a vacuum, so whatever I create has to go beyond my life. My goal is to inspire, stimulate, elicit, and encourage people to feel. I do my best to encourage everyone to be confident in themselves and their beliefs, so they will express them.

My objective has been to include and connect, and tenderly touch the hearts of everyone by sharing my vulnerabilities and challenges. I shared the many times I stumbled, not just because it's important to show that I'm human, but in the hope that others will allow themselves to become more comfortable accessing their vulnerabilities and will know there are benefits when they do. My hope is that my readers will allow themselves to feel and embrace their more sensitive sides and even share them with people whom they trust, allowing more intimate and supportive connections to be created in their lives.

Whether writing or painting, it's not uncommon for there to be moments when we feel our creation may not work out the way we thought it would. Many of us often feel like imposters who have no right calling ourselves a writer or an artist.

When a friend heard me questioning myself, to show me how ridiculous I sounded, she asked if I thought the art police were going to arrest me for being a fake. Despite this being a familiar occurrence, writers and artists still go through periods of anxiety. No matter how much talent we have or how successful we may be, we nonetheless take our self-doubts to heart.

Artists need to be aware of the light and dark throughout their paintings, while a writer is required to know where the tranquil sections are and the quickly paced or highly emotional scenes are spaced throughout her book. Artists must also be conscious of how and where color is being used while authors must "add touches of color" wherever it's needed to add depth to the manuscript—though not too little or too much.

A section of a painting may be well-painted or a scene well-written, but if it was not contributing to the painting or the book, it has to be eliminated, which is always painful.

Hours fly by when I'm writing and painting. If I stop to answer the phone, it takes a moment for my brain to engage before I can think and appropriately respond. After I'm done for the day, whether I'm writing or painting, I either feel drained or exhilarated, or some combination of the two. The work I have completed may be exactly what I want, or it may be something that needs to be trashed.

During the years I wrote this book, I kept an ongoing list of ideas to include. When I thought of something I liked, I would add it to this list.

After I finished the first draft, I read it and, if I found something intriguing or helpful, I incorporated it in the appropriate place.

These little snippets helped my book to sing. In much the same way after I would turn my almost completed artwork upside down, I could see what areas needed sharpening or where more attention was needed. Once I added these finishing touches, as if I were breathing life into it, my painting or writing lit up.

Both painting and writing require we spend much time alone. And yet after I got sick, I needed people in a way I never had before. I never would have been able to overcome what I did if hundreds of people hadn't generously given their time and shared their hearts with me. Even total strangers offered their help, and this couldn't help but change me.

Today, I feel great—emotionally, spiritually, and physically. I owe much to Dr. Deirdre O'Conner who first introduced me to natural health care. And she helped me when three neurosurgeons couldn't. I also owe a debt to Jamie Lee, DNM, IMB, who carefully listened to understand and treat my body using natural means too—along with a European Thermography test and an AO test.

By tracking my autonomic nervous system and blood flow responses, the European Thermography test detects and identifies root causes of illness *before* they become a problem. This test detects markers associated with underlying issues related to cancer years *before* a mammogram can. Despite having had breast cancer, thanks to this nonintrusive test I will never have a mammogram.

I also get an annual AO Scan from Dr. Lee, which detects abnormalities in the various energy frequencies of my cells, tissues, and organs. It resets my body's optimal frequencies to prevent disease from manifesting and restores my body to optimal health by listening to specific music the machine has chosen to help me.

No matter how frequently the radiation damage symptoms occurred, and how stubborn these symptoms were to treat, Dr. Lee never gave up on me. No longer do I get digestive or thyroid problems, heat exhaustion, problems with my hearing, or chronic fatigue syndrome. I can now usually stay up until 9:00 PM after going to bed much earlier for many years. And do I dare write this? It appears as if the damage from the radiation has finally ended because no new symptoms have surfaced for years. And thank you, Dr. Lee, for being my medical consultant on this book to make sure what I wrote was accurate.

I've worked for years to overcome the symptoms from all the traumas.

"To be honest, I'm surprised you've come as far as you have and you don't have more trauma-based symptoms," said Lynn Fraser. "When we've had experiences of feeling scared and powerless, like you have numerous times, our primitive brain and nervous system tightens, which triggers the fight/flight/freeze response. Tension builds up, and it takes time for our system to let go of all that it's been through."

"From you, Lynn, I've learned that our nervous systems are forever assessing safety and threats. And that it has a negative bias. It gives more weight to danger than safety. No wonder I've had trouble relaxing. But I've learned many resources from you that have helped me from going into survival mode, such as grounding myself by focusing on my feet, or using cyclic sighing," I said.

"Yes. None of us had resources when we were young, but as adults we can develop and strengthen our nervous system through emotional regulation," said Lynn.

This is what I've been working on for years. I now see this as an ongoing journey. I don't want any barnacles on the bottom of my boat weighing me down anymore.

Every person has the knowledge in their DNA that we won't survive without our tribe. After my family got so angry at me, I experienced this as another death threat and my body responded accordingly. Whenever I feel powerless, I now know it's because I've disconnected myself from my body and stopped listening to my heart.

Today my relationships are with people who are supportive and encourage me to be myself, with people who understand and respect my belief that when we treat ourselves and others lovingly, we align ourselves with the will of our Creator and this ignites our strength and power.

Because I chose love to guide me, I had the opportunity to experience how the world was created to support us and that we were designed to meet life wherever it is. Love played a dominant role in both the painting of the mural and the writing of this book because love became instrumental in my life, giving me the gift of empathy and compassion. I now understand love at a depth I never would have known existed. I learned that much like cockroaches, we can survive the toughest of times. The key is trusting love to guide us—and not insisting that life goes our way.

Whether you're a writer or a fine artist, a lawyer or priest, whatever it is that you do, loving yourself and sharing your love is what I recommend.

Stay connected to the love within you, so you never look outside yourself in a desperate search for love and security. Once you understand that love is within you, you'll never fear losing it because you'll know that you have the ability to create and surround yourself and feel love wherever you are.

What I succeeded in doing, and suggest to people who wish to overcome a life-threatening disease isn't easy. It's not for sissies. It's for people who are determined to become healthier and live a more fulfilling life. Because every tool I've taught you helped save my life, learning them—such as living with an open heart—will be more than worth it.

After being diagnosed with a life-threatening disease, having nervous thoughts is a typical reaction. These thoughts are generated by our nervous systems to keep us safe. But our nervous systems have memories like elephants, and they remember the times we were threatened, even when we were children, that may not be relevant today. As adults, our capacity to protect ourselves has exponentially improved.

Once you've learned to stop your emotions from hijacking you, you'll understand that for much of your life your emotions compromised your immune system and belied your reality—and disconnected you from feeling love. After you've learned to regulate your nervous system and be present in your body, you'll be able to connect within yourself again, feel secure, and think and act with maturity. And you'll see the futility of engaging with people whose emotions have hijacked them.

You'll know that you are responsible for yourself, your health and your happiness, and that freedom comes from knowing this and developing your self-awareness and this connection within yourself. Once you understand love's almighty and infinite influence, using love to heal yourself will be as natural as breathing, and that you just have to get out of your own way to feel it. And that this is when your love-filled life and healing can begin.

C. S. Lewis, one of the intellectual giants of the twentieth century said, "Experience is the most brutal of teachers, but you learn, my God, do you learn."

About the Author

Sandi Gold grew up in a seacoast town near the Connecticut-Rhode Island border, the youngest of three children. She developed artistic abilities while drawing alongside her mother, who was pursuing a master's degree in art education. Sandi earned her BFA at Boston University, and received a full scholarship to study at the Leo Marchutz School of Art in Aix-en-Provence, France.

Upon her return, Sandi moved to Washington DC, where she worked as a freelance illustrator for such clients as *The Washington Post*, The National Fisheries Association, and the Wolf Trap National Park for the Performing Arts. After her inoperable brain tumor was successfully treated, she relocated to Westerly, Rhode Island. There she opened an art studio and co-founded the Artists Cooperative of Westerly and the First Friday Westerly Arts Crawl. Her artwork has been exhibited at the Mystic Seaport Museum Maritime Art Gallery, the Mystic Museum of Art, the Newport Art Museum, and in numerous private collections.

The story of Sandi's inspirational mural, "The Temple of the Soul," was featured in *The New York Times*, *People Magazine* and ABC Television's *20/20*, where her segment was among the top three programs the year it aired. She was also interviewed on National Public Radio and its Connecticut affiliate. She was the keynote speaker for the Calgary Cancer Center in Canada and has spoken at Brown University, the Brain Tumor Society in Boston, and at schools throughout Connecticut and Rhode Island.

Sandi is a certified Expressive Arts Specialist, a certified Kripalu Holistic Teacher and a certified Kiloby Inquiries Facilitator. She has worked for area hospitals, primarily with cancer patients, using Expressive Art to assist their healing, and also for hospice as an Expressive Art Specialist.

Notably, Sandi was nominated for the National Athena Award and received a Rhode Island Citation Award and The State House of Representative Citation.

Sandi can be reached through her website www.sandigold.com, where you can also sign up for her newsletter "Love, Life & Healing."